Cognitive Behaviour Therapy for People with Intellectual Disabilities

Andrew Jahoda • Biza Stenfert Kroese
Carol Pert

Cognitive Behaviour Therapy for People with Intellectual Disabilities

Thinking creatively

palgrave
macmillan

Andrew Jahoda
Institute of Health and Wellbeing
University of Glasgow
Glasgow, UK

Biza Stenfert Kroese
School of Psychology,
University of Birmingham
Birmingham, UK

Carol Pert
Learning Disabilities Service
NHS Greater Glasgow and Clyde
Glasgow, UK

ISBN 978-1-137-47853-5   ISBN 978-1-137-47854-2 (eBook)
DOI 10.1057/978-1-137-47854-2

Library of Congress Control Number: 2017952541

© The Editor(s) (if applicable) and The Author(s) 2017
The author(s) has/have asserted their right(s) to be identified as the author(s) of this work in accordance with the Copyright, Designs and Patents Act 1988.
This work is subject to copyright. All rights are solely and exclusively licensed by the Publisher, whether the whole or part of the material is concerned, specifically the rights of translation, reprinting, reuse of illustrations, recitation, broadcasting, reproduction on microfilms or in any other physical way, and transmission or information storage and retrieval, electronic adaptation, computer software, or by similar or dissimilar methodology now known or hereafter developed.
The use of general descriptive names, registered names, trademarks, service marks, etc. in this publication does not imply, even in the absence of a specific statement, that such names are exempt from the relevant protective laws and regulations and therefore free for general use.
The publisher, the authors and the editors are safe to assume that the advice and information in this book are believed to be true and accurate at the date of publication. Neither the publisher nor the authors or the editors give a warranty, express or implied, with respect to the material contained herein or for any errors or omissions that may have been made. The publisher remains neutral with regard to jurisdictional claims in published maps and institutional affiliations.

Cover illustration: Jon Boyes/getty images

Printed on acid-free paper

This Palgrave Macmillan imprint is published by Springer Nature
The registered company is Macmillan Publishers Ltd.
The registered company address is: The Campus, 4 Crinan Street, London, N1 9XW, United Kingdom

Preface

The growth of Cognitive Behavioural Therapy (CBT) in recent years for an ever-increasing range of mental health problems has been nothing short of phenomenal, and yet people with intellectual disabilities in the UK and much of the world have missed out probably more than any other disadvantaged group in the population for help from this fast-growing development. Despite some advances, the general mind-set remains that CBT is largely inappropriate for people with intellectual disabilities, who are deemed not to have the capability to benefit from CBT. There is a widespread failure even to acknowledge that this group is especially vulnerable to mental health problems. And while there are well-intentioned national and local initiatives to improve CBT-based services, there is sadly a gulf between the rhetoric and the reality of provision on the ground. This is reflected in the fact that, while the publication of specialised CBT handbooks has flourished in virtually every other area of mental health—even areas previously also resistant to recognition as appropriate for CBT such as psychosis—there has up to now been only one book (Stenfert Kroese et al. 1997) with a uniquely service delivery-oriented and practitioner emphasis on CBT for people with intellectual disabilities. Now, two decades later than that previous book, at last we have in this book a definitive handbook for every practitioner who may work with people with intellectual disabilities.

And what a book it is. It is written by three of the UK's leading authorities in intellectual disabilities whose particular strengths lie in their unusual distinction of being immersed equally in academic and research expertise *and* clinical practice—the relatively neglected ideal of the scientist-practitioner. They thereby bring a unique depth of wisdom and breadth of scope to the application of CBT for intellectual disabilities. For here the whole range of helpers, from commissioners and planners to the individual volunteer, from seasoned practitioners to the novice, professionals and volunteers, friends and family—all will find guidance and advice honed by both years of experience and cutting-edge research. It is far beyond the scope of this brief preface to even summarise the wealth of multilayered knowledge and practical guidelines, but here are some examples to give a flavour of the points of guidance.

Firstly, the authors show that prejudiced assumptions uninformed by research evidence have led to a shocking neglect of providing CBT for people with intellectual disabilities, that people with intellectual disabilities are people who, like everyone else, want to live ordinary lives, want help with ordinary emotional and behavioural problems and, like people in general with mental health problems, can be significantly helped by CBT. Secondly, people with intellectual disabilities do *not* require a simple, dumbed-down version of CBT but precisely the same fundamentals as contained in established models of CBT, and are equally open to further third wave developments including mindfulness training. Thirdly, they stress the importance of a focused application of evidence-based CBT methods, but alongside this they utilise and develop the broader metacompetency approach, especially important in working with people with intellectual disabilities, where the therapist needs to be flexibly client-centred, drawing upon a wide range of interventions but also making creative adaptation of those approaches. The chapters that form the heart of the book outline a range of such innovations for a wide spectrum of difficulties commonly encountered in people with intellectual disabilities. Here the reader/practitioner will find chapters on the issues to consider in preparing for and starting therapy, on the first stage of therapy and developing a shared formulation, and on the middle and later stages where the focus is working towards change and problem solving, and the considerations for ending therapy.

Moving beyond traditional one-to-one therapy, the authors describe the benefits and limitations of group work, what to consider when setting up a group and how to facilitate the group, continuing the spirit of client-centredness in a setting where group dynamics are part of the equation. Another major innovation in CBT now well established is mindfulness, where the aim is not so much to change beliefs directly but to learn how to relate to them differently. The authors show how this revolutionary approach too can be applied beneficially to people with intellectual disabilities—a development perhaps even more surprising to the sceptics.

The general practice of CBT usually involves working with the client alone or in a group, with involvement of significant others only if relevant. However, in using CBT with people with intellectual disabilities, because of their greater dependence on others, most therapeutic work with this group will necessarily involve others—family, friends, and professional and voluntary care workers. The authors place particular emphasis on this unique aspect of work, and a wealth of innovative and evidence-based guidance on working with the whole range of others is provided.

I strongly recommend this book to anyone who is involved in helping people with intellectual disabilities, be they a commissioner or manager of services, a relative or friend, a professional or lay helper. There is information, guidance and advice for everyone in this comprehensive handbook, backed by research carried out by the authors and others, including the very latest findings. Despite the enormous challenge of the task, this book is optimistic, inspiring, creative and comprehensive—and sorely needed.

December 30th, 2016   Peter Trower

References

Stenfert Kroese, B., Dagnan, D., & Loumidis, K. (Eds.). (1997). *Cognitive behaviour therapy for people with learning disabilities*. London: Routledge.

To make our materials freely available to interested clinicians and researchers, we have joined a website [www.toolsfortalking.wordpress.com] that hosts a section [click on CBT—Thinking Creatively] with some of the resources that we have found useful in our work. We do not suggest that they are used exactly as they are presented, but they may function as a starting point and can be adapted to individual clients according to their needs.

Contents

1 Introduction   1

2 History and Theory   9

3 Current Context   31

4 Assessment and Setting the Scene for Cognitive Behaviour Therapy   55

5 The First Stage of Therapy   85

6 Therapeutic Change   109

7 And Another Thing… Adapting Therapy for Particular Cognitive Impairments   137

8 Group Work   157

9	Mindfulness and Third Wave Therapies	181
10	Working with Others	213
11	Making a Real Difference	237
12	Final Thoughts	255
Index		263

1

Introduction

Why Did We Write This Book?

This book provides a theoretical background to the application of Cognitive Behavioural Therapy (CBT) for people with intellectual disabilities and information on how to make this talking therapy work for these clients. We wanted to do more than write a 'cookbook' or step-by-step manual because over the years we have discovered that, although a tempting thought, people are too complex and individual for a one-recipe-fits-all approach. This type of clinical work requires flexibility, ingenuity and on-the-spot, creative problem solving on the part of the therapist. We are perhaps at risk of disappointing our readers by failing to provide them with a quick and easy guide that can be used to prepare sessions without investing much effort or time on their part. But (and we have discussed this at length), we don't want to patronise or deceive our readers and we anticipate that whoever picks up this book will aim for more thoughtful clinical practice and will have a genuine interest in the philosophical, social, psychological and political issues that provide a historical background and a current context to the therapeutic approach that we describe.

These deliberations may be considered as a frivolous luxury in this period of austerity and close health economic scrutiny. Shouldn't we all just concentrate on increasing our client contacts and stick to grabbing off-the-shelf manuals as long as these can claim to have at least some evidence base? For the three of us this has become a rhetorical question. The more we have discussed our clinical work experiences and our ideas with each other, the more obvious it has become that this type of therapeutic work cannot be reduced to a handy list of 'dos and don'ts', hence the title of this book having the subtitle 'thinking creatively', with the adverb 'creatively' defined as new, original and resourceful.

We started meeting a few years ago with the idea of writing a book that would be a timely follow-up to a book on CBT for people with intellectual disabilities that was published quite some time ago (Stenfert Kroese et al. 1997). Often referred to as 'the yellow book' (for obvious reasons), it seems to have been a helpful guide for some who, at a time when people with intellectual disabilities rarely received any talking therapies nor were sought out or listened to by researchers, had to start with an almost blank slate. The yellow book consists of a series of edited chapters by a number of early pioneer therapists and researchers who had an interest in adapting CBT for this client group and who started to believe that this could become an effective and exciting new approach. But the yellow book is now 20 years old and we have moved on, not just in CBT clinical practice but also in terms of the evidence base for talking therapies for people with intellectual disabilities.

What Position Are We Coming from?

We are all clinical psychologists who have chosen to keep one foot in clinical work and the other foot in teaching, research and writing. This allows us to inform our clinical work with our research findings while our teaching is very much based on both clinical and research experiences, and the type of research we choose to do is influenced by our clinical experiences.

We hope that this book captures some of these crossovers and that our writing conveys the belief we hold regarding the importance of providing good-quality mental health services for people with intellectual disabilities, services that acknowledge the disadvantages that many of our clients have had in their lives (and continue to experience) as well as their many strengths and positive attributes that we encounter during our therapy sessions. It goes without saying that we believe that our clients can benefit from talking therapies just as well as people with more sophisticated intellectual resources at their disposal. So from an equality as well as an efficacy perspective we see no reason why not to provide CBT for people with intellectual disabilities; to not do so would in Mike Bender's terms show a 'therapeutic distain' for people with intellectual disabilities (Bender 1993).

We must, though, acknowledge that the therapeutic work we describe in this book is limited to clients who have at least some verbal communication and we do not consider all our clients with intellectual disabilities suitable for CBT. The clients who usually receive CBT in our clinical experience are those with mild or moderate intellectual disabilities. This does not mean that we should not attempt to 'listen' to people when they cannot speak. There are ways of doing this that have an excellent evidence base whereby we can, through careful observation, come to an informed formulation (or functional analysis) of psychological and behavioural problems. We can identify what triggers adverse responses and what makes it easier for people with severe intellectual disabilities to cope with their environment. These techniques originate from the Applied Behaviour Analysis tradition and are widely and successfully used and adopted by approaches such as Durand's Functional Communication Training (Durand 1990) and more recently by Positive Behaviour Support (e.g. DOH 2014) initiatives.

We are aware that currently there are a number of terms in circulation for the particular group of people we work with and in the UK the official term that remains in common use is 'people with learning disabilities'. We have decided on 'people with intellectual disabilities' rather than 'learning disabilities' because it is a broader term and also because it is used in most English-speaking countries.

How Did We Write This Book?

Because two of us live and work in Glasgow and one in the West Midlands, we arranged to meet once every four months or so halfway down/up the railway track, in Lancaster. First we met in the intriguingly named Bashful

Alley and later in the Castle which was used as a gaol until quite recently but now has a very welcoming tearoom with large wooden tables that gave us lots of space to spread out our papers and laptops. These meetings became a highlight in our diaries and 'See you in Gaol!' became our customary cheery email sign-off message.

The discussions that took place during those meetings soon made us realise that we had many opinions and experiences in common but they also highlighted some differences. Rather than bashing away until we were in total agreement with each other and singing from exactly the same hymn sheet, we often agreed to disagree and 'respected the difference'. For example, whereas one of us listed numerous ideological and practical reasons why home visits are not a good idea for a CBT therapist, the other two argued convincingly that in certain circumstances visiting a client in their home can have benefits that outweigh the disadvantages. We spent some time trying to come to a shared view but in the end came to the considered conclusion that this book should reflect a variety of approaches and opinions and that presenting ourselves as totally in agreement on all fronts may give a false and shallow impression.

So an attentive reader will at times find slight nuances in how certain ideas and practices are described and discussed and will notice that the style and 'feel' of the chapters will vary according to who was the lead author. We are of the opinion that this is a strength of the book rather than a weakness although we are aware that with a single author, the book may have been a smoother ride for our readers.

What Is in This Book?

We anticipate that many busy clinicians and researchers will dip into this book and select just a few chapters that seem to be of most interest to them. For these readers the structure of this book is of little importance. For those who prefer to read a book from beginning to end, the structure may appear at first glance somewhat counterintuitive. What follows is an attempt at a rationale for the structure we have agreed on.

Before launching into a 'how to' account, we are keen to raise a number of issues that alert the reader to the unique aspects of this small but complex area of clinical work, some of the common pitfalls as well as an awareness of the research evidence on whether and how the CBT model can be successfully applied to people with limited intellectual functioning. So in Chap. 2 we provide our readers with a detailed account of the philosophical and historical background of CBT in general and in particular its application to people with intellectual disabilities.

Chapter 3 describes some of the current political, social and psychological context in which we as therapists attempt to deliver an effective and acceptable service to our clients. Both Chaps. 2 and 3 highlight the limitations of CBT, and of talking therapies in general, and adopt a social interactionist stance that takes account of the powerful influences, good and bad, of other people on the lives and psychological well-being of people with intellectual disabilities. Only then do we talk about the clinical application of CBT for people with intellectual disabilities, starting with assessment and then describing the early and later stages of therapy and how to end the sessions (Chaps. 4, 5 and 6). This middle section of the book uses a detailed case study that runs across all three chapters to illustrate some of the therapeutic methods and procedures. Chapter 7 was created to raise some of the common challenges that occur in therapy and describes how to address communication problems caused by memory and attention deficits and rigid thinking.

Whereas these four clinical chapters (4 to 7) are about one-to-one therapy sessions, Chap. 8 is devoted to group work and the particular benefits and challenges that this type of service delivery can produce. We then devote Chap. 9 to the exciting new 'third wave' therapies that are rapidly gaining popularity, before we introduce the topic of how to best involve other people in our therapeutic work in Chap. 10. This is an issue that is woven into the fabric of all the preceding chapters and it may seem odd to position it so late on in the book. But we made this decision because we wanted to make sure that the focus of this book first and foremost is on the clients with intellectual disabilities themselves, before we raise and discuss the needs of other stakeholders and their potential role (whether facilitating or inhibiting) in the therapeutic process.

Then we present Chap. 11 that is all about the importance of ensuring that people with intellectual disabilities have access to CBT. Unless the ideas get put into practice there is little point to this book. In contrast to the usual thinking about 'individual' therapy, we suggest that CBT should be implemented as an integrated approach, taking account of both the person and their social circumstances. By addressing organisational issues in addition to our clients' individual needs with a psychological approach, not only may our clients be enabled to improve their mental health and well-being but families, staff groups and other third parties can also be supported to maintain and generalise the progress made in the therapy sessions for the benefit not just of the clients but also for the benefit of the wider social and organisational structures in which they function. Finally, Chap. 12 is a brief glance back at the end of our journey to describe the impact this joint writing exercise has had on us and our hopes for future developments in this field, clinical progress as well as advances in relevant research, that can help us to improve our clinical skills.

Most chapters will contain some boxes in which we have sectioned off information that we consider to be relevant and complementary to the main text, yet slightly peripheral. We hope that this will allow the text to flow and also provide the reader the chance to opt in or out of such additional information.

To make our materials freely available to interested clinicians and researchers, we have joined a website (www.toolsfortalking.wordpress.com) that hosts a section (click on CBT—Thinking Creatively) with some of the materials that we have found useful in our work. We do not suggest that these materials are used exactly as they are presented, but they may function as a starting point and can be adapted to individual clients according to their needs.

What Next?

We have been influenced by many brilliant clinicians, writers and researchers, too many to mention here, but we hope that their influence will shine through what we have written (and that we have referenced their contributions properly!). We are aware that our experiences and views are often limited to the times and places specific to us. By combining our efforts in this book we hope that we have presented a somewhat wider view although we are also acutely aware that this still constitutes a narrow field in many respects and it is therefore our hope that some of our writing may inspire others to take both the clinical practice and the research to the next level.

References

Bender, M. (1993). The unoffered chair: The history of therapeutic disdain towards people with a learning disability. *Clinical Psychology Forum, 54*, 7–12.

Department of Health. (2014). *Positive and proactive care: Reducing the need for restrictive interventions*. London: Department of Health. https://www.gov.uk/government/uploads/system/uploads/attachment_data/file/300293/JRA_DoH_Guidance_on_RP_web_accessible.pdf

Durand, V. M. (1990). *Severe behavior problems: A functional communication training approach*. New York: Guilford Press.

Stenfert Kroese, B., Dagnan, D., & Loumidis, K. (Eds.). (1997). *Cognitive behaviour therapy for people with learning disabilities*. London: Routledge.

2

History and Theory

> *[W]e just talk about how to deal with our depression and anxiety and that. But she writes things, and she's doing the flipcharts. That's quite good that. She writes what you think and how you feel at the time. And how to try and cope with them, then she writes the speech bubbles. It's quite funny, she's trying to teach me how to make myself feel better.*

The quote above is from a woman who took part in a study about people with intellectual disabilities' views of Cognitive Behavioural Therapy (CBT) (Pert et al. 2012). It hints at the effort that goes into achieving change and the need to make the process meaningful and engaging. But it also begs the question about the therapist's starting point and what she is trying to achieve in the session. In this chapter we will outline a brief history of CBT and its use with people who have intellectual disabilities, and introduce some of the key underpinning theories.

Like other clinicians, we are only too aware of how challenging it can be to balance the use of theory and technique, whilst remaining flexible enough to properly acknowledge the particular needs and concerns of the people with intellectual disabilities we are working with. There is also a risk some practitioners will take the view that theory is less important when using CBT with people who have intellectual disabilities because they need to modify the approach to make it accessible. We take an opposing view and agree with Safran and Segal (1990), that to adapt an intervention, even if it is to modify the approach to make it more accessible, requires the same understanding of the underpinning theoretical model. An explicit theoretical framework gives the therapist a working model to follow and a model to share with the client and others involved with the psychotherapeutic process. Building a shared understanding of an approach like CBT helps to foster a collaborative spirit. Of course, being a CBT therapist is not just about competencies and techniques, it is also about therapists' values. The recognition that the voices of people with intellectual disabilities needed to be heard paved the way for adapting CBT for this group.

CBT: An Evolving Therapy?

The CBT-influenced interventions arising from Beck's (1976) original Cognitive Therapy (CT) and Ellis's (1973) Rational Emotive Therapy (RET) are almost too numerous to mention. These therapies include Cognitive Analytic Therapy (Ryle 1995), Compassion Focused Therapy (Gilbert and Procter 2006), Mindfulness (Segal et al. 2012) and Acceptance and Commitment Therapy (Hayes et al. 2012). Then there are a number of offshoots from the original theory that concern the adaptation of CBT for particular emotional difficulties, perhaps most notably social anxiety (Clark and Wells 1995) and psychosis (Tarrier et al. 1998). Grappling with these different strands of CBT can make it difficult to be clear about the core theory these new approaches have evolved from and the underpinning theoretical rationale.

Aaron Beck, one of the founders of CBT, wrote a paper (Beck 2005) offering a review of what had happened in the field some 40 years after he had published his first description of the approach and the underlying model. In this review he gave an account of how his ideas developed over the years. There were a number of different influences, including clinical observations from working psychoanalytically with people suffering from depression. He also found inspiration from the work of George Kelly

(1977) and Albert Ellis (1962). Kelly's personal construct theory proposed that people actively interpret and make sense of the world, building constructs of external reality that help them to negotiate their way in the world. When people develop maladaptive constructs this leads to distress. Consequently Kelly believed that therapists working with clients who are experiencing distress need to start by trying to make sense of how their clients make sense of their world. This is different from starting by trying to interpret or explain clients' actions from a particular theoretical perspective. The theory is built round the sense that the clients make of their world rather than trying to fit them into a rigid model.

Beck succinctly explained his CBT theory in terms of 'information processing' errors. In other words, people's distress is caused by their errors in interpreting the meaning of external events or internal stimuli. This can result in catastrophising or overgeneralising interpretations of events, or having a bias for particular cues. Underlying these processing errors are core schema or assumptions about oneself and the world. In Beck's original work on depression, the core schema includes 'the negative triad', with depressed individuals holding negative views about themselves, their current lives and their future. These negative self-schemas are thought to develop over time and often lie dormant, to be triggered by a particular life experience that prompts people to begin thinking in ways that are consistent with their underlying negative self-schema. The negative thoughts linked to people's negative self-schema happen automatically. Even though people may not notice these automatic thoughts or pay particular attention to them, they are thought to have an emotional impact and to play a significant role in shaping people's perceptions of events and of themselves.

Let us imagine that a core belief I hold is 'If other people don't think I am successful it means I must be a failure'. I find out at work that a colleague has been asked to apply for a post and no one has mentioned it to me. A negative thought might be that it means 'I am not good enough' and a catastrophic way of thinking about it is that 'I will never get a promotion' and that it might even mean that my manager wants 'to get rid of me because I am not good enough'. These core beliefs help to shape people's perceptions of events. Crucially, negative interpretations of the events, rather than the events themselves, cause distress. Where the behavioural component comes in is that people's actions are also linked to their interpretations of events. For example, a woman with an intellectual disability in supported employment may lack confidence and come to believe that her supervisor is unhappy with the job she's doing and think she is a 'failure'. Consequently, she might try to avoid her supervisor. The problem with this strategy is that the lack of evidence to the contrary just helps to confirm the negative beliefs that she holds about herself. Avoiding her supervisor means that she has even less chance of finding out what he really thinks about her. Also, her avoidant behaviour may give a negative impression and result in her supervisor actually thinking less well of her.

CBT works by attempting to help people to become aware of and change unhelpful thinking patterns and, in doing so, reduce their distress and help them to bring their lives back on track. The aim is to help the person to challenge the thoughts or underlying schemas that lead to their distress and to practise different ways of thinking about and negotiating their world. The assumption is that the therapist and client will work collaboratively to achieve this goal. This is not only for the purpose of building rapport and a successful relationship with the client but also because the idea is to lead the client on a journey of 'guided self-discovery'. The therapist is not revealing truths but is helping the clients to find for themselves different and more adaptive ways of thinking and behaving. For this reason, Socratic questioning is used, a way of helping people to reflect on their thinking without trying to impose a different view in a didactic way. Self-monitoring and behavioural experiments are then used to check out whether particular ways of thinking really do cause them problems in their everyday lives. In the example given above, the worker in supported employment was worried that her supervisor thought she was doing a bad job. In therapy she might have rated her work performance as 1 out of 5. A behavioural experiment, with the help of her job coach, might have involved asking her supervisor to rate her work. If she found out that her work was rated by her supervisor as 4 out of 5, this might have helped to change her perceptions. Consequently, the aim is to have an impact on not only people's cognitions but also the lives that they lead.

Interestingly, Beck did not just jump straight to outcome trials to examine whether or not CBT proved to be effective; he began by exploring whether the ideas underpinning his therapy were correct. In other words, he wanted to know if his insights and observations and the theories he developed really reflected the nature of depressed people's thinking and beliefs. So he was not merely content to find out if the therapy worked, but he was also interested in research investigating whether the beliefs and thinking styles of individuals with depression fitted with the model he proposed. In a similar vein, when CBT was developed to address social anxiety, the intervention was influenced by an attempt to understand the nature of socially anxious people's difficulties. Clark and Wells's (1995) model takes account of the finding that people experiencing social anxiety become absorbed by their distressing thoughts and preoccupied by how they are viewed by others. This inward focus on their distress heightens their somatic symptoms of anxiety. Consequently, they may be even more reluctant to actually engage with other people in case their worst fears about people judging them negatively are confirmed. Not only is this distressing at the time but it might leave them with an upsetting memory. Clark and Well's model of social anxiety shows that CBT cannot simply be applied to different problem areas as a set of processes. A crucial starting point is to ensure that the particular approach taken to address people's problems makes sense to them, both in terms of how they perceive internal and external stimuli and in how they negotiate their world.

Albert Ellis was the founder of Rational Emotive Behavioural Therapy (REBT), a strand of CT that predated Beck's model. He also proposed that the way people think about or interpret events mediates their emotional reactions and that their interpretations of events are linked to maladaptive assumptions they hold about themselves and their world (Ellis 1962). A number of ideas from REBT will be included in this book, as we believe that they lend themselves well to working with people who have intellectual disabilities. The ABC model, where the A represents the **a**ctivating events, B represents the **b**eliefs or interpretations about the events and C the emotional and behavioural **c**onsequences, offers a clear framework that can be shared with clients. By promoting the use of active tasks in therapy, such as role play and getting clients to practise using positive self-statements, REBT can help to make the therapeutic process more accessible and alive for clients (Bernard, Ellis and Terjerson, 2006) and this is particularly relevant for our clients with intellectual disabilities.

The Evidence

In 2006 Beck also published a meta-analysis of meta-analyses of studies concerning the use of CBT for 14 emotional and interpersonal problem areas (Butler et al. 2006). This review of review papers, pulling together all the available evidence, concerned clinical trials for a remarkable range of therapies for mental health problems including depression, social phobia, psychosis and interventions for anger and offending. Nevertheless, a noteworthy exclusion criterion for taking part in any of the 332 studies was having an intellectual disability. It is probably fair to say that within the mainstream adult mental health therapeutic community there is a continuing scepticism about the use of CBT with people who have intellectual disabilities. Clearly, CBT is a talking therapy that is not accessible to all people who have an intellectual disability. But it is puzzling why CBT should be considered to be inappropriate for such a heterogeneous group, especially for those with mild disabilities. Scoring a few less IQ points on a psychometric test does not make someone a distinctly different kind of person. Taylor et al. (2008) drew on the small existing evidence base to contest the 'therapeutic disdain' (Bender 1993) that has often resulted in people with intellectual disabilities being excluded from psychological therapies such as CBT. However, it is true that CBT is only accessible to a proportion of people with intellectual disabilities and Chaps. 4 and 5 will consider ways of helping to determine whether CBT is potentially appropriate and accessible for them.

Early groundbreaking case studies point to the potential effectiveness of CBT for people with intellectual disabilities (see Stenfert Kroese et al. 1997), and offer important guidance to clinicians about how CBT can be adapted. CBT has now been adapted for use with people who have an intellectual disability and a range of additional difficulties, including anxiety, psychosis, trauma and sex offending (Taylor et al. 2008). This pioneering work has paved the way for a number of clinical trials, allowing researchers to say with more confidence that CBT can be an effective way of helping people with intellectual disabilities with emotional and/or interpersonal difficulties.

Vereenooghe and Langdon (2013) carried out a meta-analysis of controlled studies of psychological therapies for people with intellectual disabilities. In other words, to be included in their meta-analysis the studies had to compare the outcomes of people receiving a psychological therapy like CBT with a control group of some description. Vereenooghe and Langdon concluded from their analyses that CBT for anger and depression was moderately effective.

This emerging evidence is promising but with 11 of the 15 CBT studies concerning anger management, it leads to a number of other questions about the use of CBT with people who have intellectual disabilities. Anger management only accounts for one small area of work in the wider general adult mental health field (Butler et al. 2006). One reason for this difference may be that people with intellectual disabilities rarely refer themselves for help with their emotional or interpersonal difficulties. Someone else usually refers them for help, often because their difficulties have become a problem for others. Anger problems may, therefore, be a common outward sign of emotional distress that results in a referral to services. Being referred by someone else has major implications for how people perceive therapy and even whether they believe they need help at all. People's expectations and beliefs about therapy and the implications for engagement and outcome will be discussed in Chaps. 4 and 5.

Deficits and Distortions

Another possible explanation for the large number of CBT anger management studies is that this is a particularly apt intervention for people with intellectual disabilities. It has been argued that some of the main components of anger management work address 'cognitive deficits' rather than the 'cognitive distortions' or errors that Beck made the focus of his original CT intervention for depression (Jahoda et al. 2001). Using an 'information processing' approach to explain psychological distress with people who have intellectual disabilities is complicated by the fact that, by definition, they already have cognitive impairments. This means that the distress they experience with understanding and negotiating their world could be attributed to their intellectual disabilities. For example, people with anger problems might be more likely to perceive someone else's actions as threatening if they have difficulties interpreting others' actions or emotions. They may also be more likely to respond in an aggressive way if they have limited problem-solving skills, have difficulty with emotional regulation or find it difficult to think through the consequences of their actions. Self-talk or inner speech is said to play a vital role in helping people to coordinate and employ any new cognitive skills and strategies that they may learn in therapy, and to apply them in novel settings (Meichenbaum and Asarnow 1978; Bernard et al. 2006). However, the idea of self-instructional training begs the question about who the self is that one is training?

A client needs to be motivated to change or to be at least interested in acquiring new skills if they are going to change their behaviour or gain greater emotional control. In turn, learning more adaptive ways of coping with situations that previously led to conflict with other people is likely to change the dynamic of the situation and the client's view of other people and themselves (Bernard et al. 2009). Thus, the process of change when a client learns self-regulation skills or new coping mechanisms may be less mechanistic than appears at first sight and it may be misleading to categorise or compartmentalise the different components of therapy as 'cognitive' or 'behavioural'. Even if it is the case that a great deal of 'cognitive therapy' carried out with clients who have intellectual disabilities has actually been concerned with cognitive and behavioural deficits, potentially linked to their intellectual disabilities (Willner 2006), the underlying aim remains to increase the person's agency and foster an awareness that different ways of negotiating their world can improve their sense of well-being.

Compared to cognitive deficits, much less attention has been paid to our clients' possible misinterpretations of the world (cognitive distortions). These abstract issues, such as the link between clients' interpretations of events and their resulting feelings and behaviour, are more complex to tackle in therapy (Bernard et al. 2006). Then there is the even trickier task of helping clients to generalise the skills and insights gained in therapy sessions to everyday life. Receptive and expressive verbal understanding, memory, abstract reasoning and planning are just some of the cognitive abilities that might be tested in the course of therapy. This book will draw on the existing body of literature and clinical observation and experience to describe how CBT can be adapted to take account of clients' cognitive difficulties so as to access and challenge cognitive distortions.

Quite apart from people's cognitive difficulties, another reason why less attention has been paid to the mediating role of cognitive distortions is because, in reality, people with intellectual disabilities face considerable challenges in real life that have an impact on their emotional well-being. Real frustrations stem from having difficulty managing everyday demands, such as tasks that involve literacy or numeracy. There are also the social consequences of having an intellectual disability and belonging to a stigmatised group, which might include being bullied, excluded or overprotected by those who love you (Cooney et al. 2006). In practical terms, this means that the therapeutic models might need to be subtly adapted. For example, Clark and Wells' CBT approach to social anxiety begins with the premise that people make errors about how they are being judged by other people. Consequently, a key aim of their intervention is to help the person to pay more attention to external reality, to counteract their irrational beliefs that other people are watching them and judging them in ways that make them feel humiliated. But what if the truth is that other people are staring at them or judge them negatively as a person because they have an intellectual disability? Highly distressing attributions might arise from realistic appraisals people make about their social circumstances and treatment by others, including being stigmatised and socially excluded. Perhaps in these circumstances the focus needs to be shifted onto people's secondary appraisals, to help them retain a positive sense of self in the face of such threats. It may be that for people with intellectual disabilities, CBT is not always about shifting people's distorted perceptions about the external world but about how they come to perceive and value themselves. Working with the evaluations (secondary appraisals) people make about themselves, rather than challenging the inferences they make about what is actually happening, is a well-established approach in REBT (Trower et al. 2015). Of course, there also needs to be a focus on the environment, to help tackle the ill treatment people experience or to promote real opportunities for social inclusion.

Just as Beck found for the general clinical population, it is important to note that there is evidence about the influence of people with intellectual disabilities' attributions or interpretation of events on their emotional reactions and interpersonal perceptions. Esbensen and Benson (2004) showed that negative automatic thoughts and feelings of helplessness were associated with depressive symptoms reported by people with mild intellectual disabilities. Similarly, the role of cognitive factors has been demonstrated in the field of anger and aggression. Jahoda et al. (2006) found that aggressive individuals made similar attributions of hostile intent as their non-aggressive peers when observing others facing provocation. However, when they were asked to imagine themselves facing provocation the pattern changed. In this self-referent condition the aggressive individuals attributed higher levels of hostile intent to the provocateur than their non-aggressive peers. If the participants' problems of aggression had simply been due to a lack of socio-emotional understanding or deficient rule-governed behaviour, then they would have been expected to perceive a higher level of hostile intent irrespective of whether they were observing others or imagining that they were facing threat themselves. Instead, the meaning and context of the event appears to be crucial to how people interpret particular situations and to their subsequent feelings and actions. This highlights the potential value of adopting cognitive interventions that move beyond an educational or self-regulatory approach, and that investigate and aim to modify thoughts and beliefs specific to the individual client.

Making Therapy Meaningful: Asking the Right Questions

A challenge for us when considering the meaning our clients attach to their experiences is that their concerns may not always be explicit or fully expressed. This can happen for a host of reasons, including a sense of shame about talking about particular topics or because some topics are taboo. This can be even more challenging if people have difficulty with expressive language and putting their views across or have problems with inter-subjectivity. In other words, they may have a tendency to assume that their therapist knows the characters, background or circumstances being talked about. This means that it is important for the therapist to be alive to the kind of things that people might become depressed, distressed or anxious about. For example, it is remarkable how often people's disability itself can be a topic that is, in classic counselling parlance, the elephant in the room that is rarely mentioned.

Care must be taken to avoid perceiving people with intellectual disabilities as a different kind of people. They are socialised into the same world as their non-disabled peers and face the same slings and arrows, and highs and lows, including bereavement, loss and trauma. The aim of taking account of the past experiences of people with an intellectual disability is not to characterise their lives as all tragedy or trauma. Rather, it is simply to acknowledge that the real challenges people face and the meaning they attach to events influence their emotional experiences and ultimately their mental health. In turn, the specific challenges that our clients with intellectual disabilities are likely to experience have implications for how CBT is adapted for them. But we should also remember that many people with intellectual disabilities can and do lead fulfilling lives. Retaining a sense of what is possible is vital, if the aim of the work is not merely to counter clients' maladaptive patterns of thinking and behaving but also to build on their strengths. This was a subject that social scientists were concerned with in the past, at a time when there was a shift away from deterministic views about the impact of having an intellectual disability. Robert Edgerton's (1967) anthropological study of people leaving a long stay hospital in the 1960s USA remains a classic text, with remarkable insights into the struggle of living with a stigmatised identity. Whilst a significant number of people Edgerton followed up faced the harsh realities of living in desperate poverty, the remarkable resilience and resourcefulness shown by many was striking.

People with intellectual disabilities continue to face distinct challenges and it is important for therapists to be aware of these as possible sources of distress. An example of how such insights might be helpful can be illustrated by a piece of research carried out by Marisa Forte who compared the worries of young college students with intellectual disabilities and their non-disabled peers (Forte et al. 2011). Interestingly, the main worries identified by the two groups were distinctly different. While the young people with intellectual disabilities said that their main worries were about being bullied, death, failure and friendships, the young people without intellectual disabilities said they were most concerned about getting a job, money, failure and making decisions. In the one area of overlap between the groups, worry about failure, there was a distinct difference in the content of the worries that were reported. Whereas the non-disabled young people worried about failing their exams or driving tests, those with intellectual disabilities worried about a more general sense of failing to achieve expected life goals like getting a job or parenthood. There was a sense that those without disabilities were most worried about coping with specific future responsibilities and opportunities, while those with disabilities were more concerned about a general lack of future opportunities and adult roles.

The finding that people with intellectual disabilities were worried about death came from a fear of losing a family carer. Moving towards adulthood seemed to have made these young people aware of their dependence on others for help and made them increasingly anxious about who would be there to support them in the longer term. The young people without a disability who expressed worry about death were concerned with their own mortality.

No one in Forte's study was receiving help for clinically significant emotional problems. Nevertheless, the contrasting reports by the young people with and without intellectual disabilities offers an insight into the ways that different life experiences and circumstances shaped their outlooks. The need to take time to explore the content of clients' concerns and to be aware of their particular life experiences and personal histories will be carefully considered in Chaps. 4, 5 and 6. A crucial starting point is for therapists to have the sensitivity and insight to ask the right questions.

Therapy in Context

One of the main criticisms of using approaches like CBT with the general population is that it risks scapegoating individuals for wider social problems (Moloney and Kelly 2004). If you are poor, socially marginalised or have been abused in the past then you are more likely to experience mental health problems or emotional distress (Marmot 2005). More recently, people like Eric Emerson and Chris Hatton have pointed to social causes of emotional distress experienced by people with intellectual disabilities like poverty, social exclusion and bullying (Emerson 2010; Emerson and Hatton 2007; Emerson et al. 2014). They refer to these causes as 'upstream', meaning that these broader social factors or circumstances are major contributory factors to individuals' mental health problems. At a time of increasing austerity and discussions about the role of the state in supporting its most vulnerable citizens, the broader social and service contexts cannot be ignored by therapists when considering the limits and potential of an individual psychotherapeutic approach like CBT.

Yet when it comes to working with people who have intellectual disabilities and are presenting with emotional problems, there has been a long-standing tradition of taking the impact of their wider environment seriously (Clements 1997). In the past, this has been linked to an awareness of the damaging and depersonalising impact of institutional environments. Recent events showing the harrowing treatment of people living in some of our present-day institutions (Department of Health 2012) suggests that much more needs to be done to prevent cultures of abuse causing dreadful damage to people's lives. Those working therapeutically in community settings continue to take clients' broader life circumstances seriously. This is not just as background factors to take into consideration for a psychological formulation (see Chap. 5) to help shape the individual therapy, but working with people's life circumstances becomes the stuff of therapy itself. Engaging with clients' broader lives helps to make a therapeutic approach like CBT more meaningful and relevant. For one thing, therapists need to be sensitive and aware of the reality of people's lives because clients' concerns are not merely a set of symptoms but instead are thoughts expressed in relation to the lives that they lead or want to lead. In their response to the new version of the Diagnostic and Statistical Manual of Mental Disorders, Fifth Edition (DSM-V) (American Psychiatric Association 2013), the British Psychological Society made a number of telling criticisms. These criticisms included a quote from Peter Beresford about the risk of marginalising lived experience when using diagnostic classification systems for mental health problems:

> Service users often emphasise the primary significance of practical, material, interpersonal and social aspects of their experiences, which only constitute

subsidiary or 'trigger' factors in the current system of classification. (Beresford 2013)

The interpersonal and social aspects of clients' experiences take on a particular significance if they are socially marginalised and remain dependent upon others for support in aspects of everyday life. Chapter 10 considers ways of working alongside organisations, staff and family members using CBT interventions. Helping clients to negotiate and maintain change means working with those who will continue to play a crucial role in clients' lives long after the therapists have gone.

A Theoretical Framework: The Social Self

The information processing approach proposed by Beck (1976) and Ellis (1973) has a focus on individual agency and changing how individuals think about and behave in the world. In keeping with an interest in the wider context of people's lives, we want to draw on symbolic interactionist theories of the self, to consider how people with limited ability to achieve change in their own right can be supported to do so. Symbolic interactionist theories (Mead 1934) propose that people's sense of self does not exist in a vacuum. As the Scottish enlightenment philosopher Adam Smith explained:

> Were it possible that a human creature could grow up to manhood in a solitary place, without any communication with his one species, he could no more think of his own character or the propriety or demerits of his sentiments and conduct, or the beauty of his own mind, than of the beauty or deformity of his own face. All these are objects which he cannot easily see ... and with regard to which he is provided with no mirror which can present them to his view. Bring him into society, and he is immediately provided with the mirror he wanted before. (Smith 1759/1976, p. 110)

Mead suggested that our sense of who we are is, at least in part, shaped by how others respond to us or the mirror they hold up to us. Clearly, not everyone's views have the same impact and the views of significant others; our parents, in particular, play the most important role as we grow up.

We also internalise a model of how the social world works or a sense of the 'generalised other'. Thankfully, having an internalised model of how the social world works also allows us to learn through reflecting upon our actions and means that we are not trapped by our social circumstances. It is also possible for us to act in ways that are surprising or novel.

We use symbolic interactionist theory to extend the CBT model for working with people who have an intellectual disability. That is, when we are working therapeutically with clients using CBT, we are not just trying to change unhelpful thinking patterns. By helping clients to overcome distress or destructive patterns of interpersonal behaviour, we are hoping that they can make real change in their lives. This might mean someone who presented with significant anger problems is able to enjoy better relationships with others or someone who has been highly socially anxious is able to go out to social settings that they previously avoided. But what happens when the anxious person finds it difficult to make new relationships because they are socially marginalised or when others fail to acknowledge that the person with anger management problems has changed? Helping someone to make new social contacts or encouraging others to recognise that someone has changed can also help to shift our clients' self-perceptions. We have found that involving others in our therapeutic work can be a powerful way of influencing clients' self and interpersonal perceptions. People's cognitive processes are not 'sealed off' but reflect their dynamic relationship with the world in which they live.

There are also pragmatic reasons for including 'significant others' in the therapeutic process. People who have intellectual disabilities are usually more reliant on others for support with everyday decisions and tasks. This means that other people may have an important role to play both in the therapeutic process and in helping people to maintain or build on the progress they have made in therapy. For example, graded exposure may be planned as part of an intervention for someone with anxiety problems. This might involve a visit to a shopping centre and it may be necessary to enlist the help of a support worker to accompany the person to travel on public transport. However, the involvement of 'significant others' is not always straightforward. There may be tensions between a wish to ensure meaningful change happens in someone's life by enlisting the support of someone else and the client's wish to develop a confiding therapeutic relationship with their therapist. There is no one right answer about whether or not significant others should be included in a person's therapy. This is a key issue that will be addressed in more detail in Chap. 8 and it is hoped that this will help clinicians to decide when to include significant others in therapy and how best to manage this.

Therapeutic Sessions: An Interpersonal Process

Another core theme of this book concerns the importance of the therapeutic relationship. Relationships are the central ingredient of therapeutic sessions (Duncan et al. 2010) and establishing a collaborative approach between the therapist and the client is the cornerstone of CBT. There has been a growing interest in the part played by these 'non-specific' factors in therapy change in the general adult mental health field. It is surprising how little attention this topic has received in work with people who have intellectual disabilities. As therapists, we know that a good therapeutic relationship is an essential building block for CBT and working collaboratively. This way of working is not always easy to establish when the client, due to their intellectual disability, remains uncertain about what CBT is or what they want to achieve from therapy.

Key concepts from Vygotsky's work (Reiber and Robinson 2004) may help to provide a basis for the adaptations to CBT that are required for working alongside people with an intellectual disability. We are not the first to suggest that Vgotsky's constructs, such as the 'zone of proximal development', are helpful when building an engaging and meaningful therapeutic process. Paul Chadwick (2006) has offered a convincing argument for the use of Vygotsky's approach when using CBT with people who have a diagnosis of psychosis. The concept of 'zone of proximal development' proposes that people can learn more effectively in collaboration with others, when another more expert person provides support to help 'scaffold' their thinking. Importantly, the notion of scaffolding suggests that people's potential is not restricted by the level of their internal resources alone, but also by their ability to develop their thinking in dialogue with others. It requires the therapist to establish a collaborative dialogue that the client can engage in. To do this, the therapist needs to begin with a clear idea of what the client is thinking because to scaffold change means starting where the client 'is at', not in a void. The other key component of scaffolding that perhaps extends the theoretical position of Beck (1976) is that it moves beyond the idea that Socratic questioning is necessarily the key way of helping people to correct thinking errors. What if people find it difficult to generate alternative ways of thinking, as many people with intellectual disabilities do? Allowing scaffolding means that the therapist can bring to the dialogue views and suggestions about adaptive ways of thinking and behaving that the client would not be able to generate or consider as new strategies to try out.

Conclusions

As stated at the outset, CBT is a dynamic approach with a myriad of related offshoots, theories and techniques. This can lead to some cynicism, or alternatively a view in some quarters that CBT is a panacea for all ills. The aims for this book though are relatively modest, to guide the reader to adapt and deliver some of the key elements of CBT for people with intellectual disabilities. We are only too aware of the excitement amongst colleagues working with people with intellectual disabilities about the potential benefits of Mindfulness-based approaches (Chapman et al. 2013). For this reason, Chap. 9 of this book will look at these emerging strands of work and consider their implications for delivering CBT to people with intellectual disabilities.

We also hope that the reader will not regard the account given in the book as merely a simplified form of CBT for people with cognitive difficulties. The adaptations that are described draw on values and a theoretical framework that we believe have something to add to thinking in the field. People with intellectual disabilities are a socially marginalised group who remain reliant on the support of others. In this context, CBT cannot simply be about individual change and self-determined efforts to overcome distress, it also has to address people's social circumstances and what support or relationships the person might need to sustain well-being in the longer term. In the next chapter we will argue for *meta-competent adherence* (Whittington and Grey 2014) to the CBT model to make it accessible and meaningful to our clients and so have a real impact on their psychological well-being.

> **Key Points**
> - Adapted CBT is a talking therapy and individuals will need sufficient receptive expressive verbal ability to engage in the therapy and talk about their thoughts and feelings.
> - There is promising evidence about the adaptation of CBT for people with intellectual disabilities.
> - Adapted therapy should be based on a thorough understanding of the CBT model.
> - The cognitive element of CBT should not only focus on cognitive deficits relating to clients' intellectual impairments but also the meaning they attach to events and the cognitive errors and distortions they make.
> - Therapy should also concern the nature of the clients' self-perceptions or evaluations of self.
> - Adapted CBT needs to take account of the life circumstances of people with intellectual disabilities.

References

American Psychiatric Association. (2013). *Diagnostic and statistical manual of mental disorders* (5th ed.). Arlington: American Psychiatric Publishing.

Beck, A. T. (1976). *Cognitive therapy and the emotional disorders*. New York: International Universities Press.

Beck, A. T. (2005). The current state of cognitive therapy: A 40-year retrospective. *Archives of General Psychiatry, 62*, 953–959.

Bender, M. (1993). The unoffered chair: The history of therapeutic disdain towards people with a learning disability. *Clinical Psychology Forum, 54*, 7–12.

Beresford, P. (2013). Experiential knowledge and the reconception of madness. In S. Coles, S. Keenan, & B. Diamond (Eds.), *Madness contested: Power and practice*. Ross-on-Wye: PCCS Books.

Bernard, M. E., Ellis, A., & Terjersen, M. (2006). Rational emotive behavioral approaches to childhood disorders: History, theory, practice, and research. In M. Bernard & A. Ellis (Eds.), *Rational emotive behavioral approaches to childhood disorders: Theory, practice, and research* (pp. 3–84). New York: Springer.

Butler, A. C., Chapman, J. E., Forman, E. M., & Beck, A. T. (2006). The empirical status of cognitive-behavioral therapy: A review of meta-analyses. *Clinical Psychology Review, 26*, 17–31.

Chadwick, P. (2006). *Person based cognitive theory for distressing psychosis.* Chichester: Wiley.

Chapman, M. J., Hare, D. J., Caton, S., Donalds, D., McInnis, E., & Mitchell, D. (2013). The use of mindfulness with people with intellectual disabilities: A systematic review and narrative analysis. *Mindfulness, 4*, 1–11.

Clark, D. M., & Wells, A. (1995). A cognitive model of social phobia. In M. Liebowitz & R. G. Heimberg (Eds.), *Social phobia: Diagnosis, assessment, and treatment* (pp. 69–93). New York: Guilford Press.

Clements, J. (1997). Sustaining a cognitive psychology for people with learning disabilities. In B. Stenfert Kroese, D. Dagnan, & K. Lumidis (Eds.), *Cognitive behaviour therapy for people with learning disabilities* (pp. 162–181). London: Routledge.

Cooney, G., Jahoda, A., Gumley, A., & Knott, F. (2006). Young people with learning disabilities attending mainstream and segregated schooling: Perceived stigma, social comparisons and future aspirations. *Journal of Intellectual Disability Research, 50*, 432–445.

Department of Health. (2012). *Transforming care: A national response to winterbourne view hospital.* Whitehall: Department of Health.

Duncan, B. L., Miller, S. D., Wampold, B. E., & Hubble, M. A. (2010). *The heart and soul of change: Delivering what works in therapy* (2nd ed.). Washington, DC: American Psychological Association.

Edgerton, R. B. (1967). *The cloak of competence.* Berkeley: University of California Press.

Ellis, A. (1962). *Reason and emotion in psychotherapy.* New York: Norton.

Ellis, A. (1973). *Humanistic psychotherapy.* New York: McGraw-Hill.

Emerson, E. (2010). Self-reported exposure to disablism is associated with poorer self-reported health and well-being among adults with intellectual disabilities in England: A cross-sectional survey. *Public Health, 124*(12), 682–689.

Emerson, E., & Hatton, C. (2007). The contribution of socio-economic position to the health inequalities faced by children and adolescents with intellectual disabilities in Britain. *American Journal of Mental Retardation, 112*(2), 140–150.

Emerson, E., Hatton, C., Robertson, J., & Baines, S. (2014). Perceptions of neighborhood quality, social and civic participation and the self-rated health of British adults with intellectual disability: Cross sectional study. *BMC Public Health, 14*, 1252.

Esbensen, A. J., & Benson, B. A. (2004). Cognitive variables and depressed mood in adults with intellectual disability. *Journal of Intellectual Disability Research, 49*, 481–489.

Forte, M., Jahoda, A., & Dagnan, D. (2011). An anxious time? Exploring the nature of worries experienced by young people with a mild to moderate intellectual disability as they make the transition to adulthood. *British Journal of Clinical Psychology, 50*(4), 398–411.

Gilbert, P., & Procter, S. (2006). Compassionate mind training for people with high shame and self-criticism: Overview and pilot study of a group therapy approach. *Clinical Psychology & Psychotherapy, 13*, 353–379.

Hayes, S. C., Strosahl, K. D., & Wilson, K. G. (2012). *Acceptance and commitment therapy: The process and practice of mindful change* (2nd ed.). New York: The Guilford Press.

Jahoda, A., Trower, P., Pert, C., & Fin, D. (2001). Contingent reinforcement or defending the self? A review of evolving models of aggression in people with mild learning disabilities. *British Journal of Medical Psychology, 74*, 305–321.

Jahoda, A., Pert, C., & Trower, P. (2006). Frequent aggression and attribution of hostile intent in people with mild to moderate mental retardation: An empirical investigation. *American Journal on Mental Retardation, 111*(2), 90–99.

Kelly, G. A. (1977). Personal construct theory and the psychotherapeutic interview. *Cognitive Therapy and Research, 1*(4), 355–362.

Marmot, M. (2005). Social determinants of health inequalities. *Lancet, 365*(9464), 1099–1104.

Mead, G. H. (1934). *Mind, self and society.* Chicago: University of Chicago Press.

Meichenbaum, D., & Asarnow, J. (1978). Cognitive behavioral modification and metacognitive development: Implications for the classroom. In P. Kendall & S. Hollon (Eds.), *Cognitive behavioral interventions: Theory, research, and procedure* (pp. 11–35). New York: Academic.

Moloney, P., & Kelly, P. (2004). Beck never lived in Birmingham: Why CBT may be a less useful treatment for psychological distress than is often supposed. *Clinical Psychology, 34*, 4–10.

Pert, C., Jahoda, A., Stenfert Kroese, B., Trower, P., Dagnan, D., & Selkirk, M. (2012). Cognitive behavioural therapy from the perspective of clients with mild intellectual disabilities: A qualitative investigation of process issues. *Journal of Intellectual Disability Research, 57*, 359–369.

Reiber, R. W., & Robinson, D. K. (Eds.). (2004). *The essential Vygotsky.* New York: Plenum.

Ryle, A. (1995). *Cognitive analytic therapy: Developments in theory and practice*. Chichester: Wiley.

Safran, J. D., & Segal, Z. V. (1990). *Cognitive therapy: An interpersonal process perspective*. New York: Basic Books.

Segal, Z. V., Williams, J. M. G., & Teasdale, J. D. (2012). *Mindfulness-based cognitive therapy for depression*. London: Guilford Press.

Smith, A. (1759). *The theory of moral sentiments* (Republished 1976 ed.). Oxford: Clarendon Press.

Stenfert Kroese, B., Dagnan, D., & Loumidis, K. (Eds.). (1997). *Cognitive behaviour therapy for people with learning disabilities*. London: Routledge.

Tarrier, N., Yusupoff, L., Kinney, C., McCarthy, E., Gledhill, A., Haddock, G., & Morris, J. (1998). Randomised controlled trial of intensive cognitive behaviour therapy for patients with chronic schizophrenia. *British Medical Journal, 317*, 303–307.

Taylor, J. L., Lindsay, W. R., & Willner, P. (2008). CBT for people with intellectual disabilities: Emerging evidence, cognitive ability and IQ effects. *Behavioural and Cognitive Psychotherapy, 36*, 723–733.

Trower, P., Jones, J., & Dryden, W. (2015). *Cognitive-Behavioural counselling in action* (3rd ed.). London: Sage.

Vereenooghe, L., & Langdon, P. E. (2013). Psychological therapies for people with intellectual disabilities: A systematic review and meta-analysis. *Research in Developmental Disabilities, 34*(11), 4085–4102.

Whittington, A., & Grey, N. (2014). *How to become a more effective CBT therapist*. Chichester: Wiley.

Willner, P. (2006). The effectiveness of psychotherapeutic interventions for people with learning disabilities: A critical overview. *Journal of Intellectual Disability Research, 49*, 73–85.

3

Current Context

To consider how clinicians can introduce CBT to people with intellectual disabilities, we will use this chapter 'to set the scene' and to describe and discuss the service context, why people with intellectual disabilities are in need of talking therapies such as CBT, how CBT services are best accessed and the challenges that therapists may encounter. We will touch on some approaches and conceptual frameworks that we have found helpful in this context. In particular, we consider the concept of *metacompetent adherence* (Whittington and Grey (2014) useful to avoid becoming unfocused and 'drifting' to a watered-down version of CBT that is no longer evidence based and less likely to be effective. The specific techniques that we have adopted and developed will be discussed in later chapters; this current chapter will touch on broader context and political and clinical issues.

Service Responses to People with Intellectual Disabilities and Mental Health Problems

The UK Equality Act 2010 states that it is the duty of public organisations to reduce inequalities that may arise for people with 'protected characteristics', which includes people with disabilities and therefore also people with intellectual disabilities. On the basis of this in England the 'Improving Access to Psychological Therapies' (IAPT) programme aims to address inequalities by:

> expanding access to NICE approved psychological therapies across all communities particularly for people that are at higher risk of developing poor mental health due to social, economic and health inequalities (Department of Health, 2011).

People with intellectual disabilities certainly fall into the category of *'people that are at higher risk of developing poor mental health due to social, economic and health inequalities'*. If challenging behaviour and autistic spectrum disorders are included, over 40% of the adult population with intellectual disabilities were found to have additional mental health needs by one group of researchers (Cooper et al. 2007). Yet, whilst researching for this book in September 2016 we found that the page 'Learning Difficulties' on the IAPT (Improving Access to Psychological Therapies) website (www.iapt.nhs.uk) was a blank. Although the client group was considered to be important enough to create a separate website page, unlike the 'Older People' page, no one had as yet made an effort to collate information about intellectual disabilities initiatives or statistics on access to treatment, effectiveness or specialist training, which may say something about how seriously the equality agenda was taken.

Why Such High Prevalence of Mental Health Problems?

When people with intellectual disabilities have mental health problems, the causes are often linked to the difficulties that people encounter as a result of their disabilities. For example, being highly dependent on others and having limited opportunities to make choices can prevent people from developing self-esteem or self-acceptance, a sense that their life is worth living and a belief that the future holds interesting and achievable challenges. Meaningful relationships are often lacking for adults with intellectual disabilities, and very few are able to develop typical adult roles of paid worker, consumer, sexual partner or parent in their lifetime. That is, they will rarely achieve the positions in life that provide most adults with positive, albeit at times stressful, experiences. Not being able to take on such meaningful and valued roles in adult life is likely to increase vulnerability to low mood and a host of mental health problems, especially depression and anxiety.

As is the case for the rest of the population, trauma and abuse (including physical, sexual, financial and emotional abuse) are also reasons why people with intellectual disabilities may suffer psychological problems, particularly psychotic symptoms such as hearing voices or heaving chronic delusions. Rates of sexual and physical abuse across the life span are higher for people with intellectual disabilities (Lindsay et al. 2006) because of high dependency on others and difficulties in recognising and reporting abuse. This may account for the finding that the prevalence rates for the diagnosis of, for example, schizophrenia have been reported to be three times higher than expected (e.g. Morgan et al. 2008). Other common presenting problems for people exposed to traumatic events include typical PTSD (posttraumatic stress disorder) symptoms such as anxiety, flashbacks and recurring nightmares, as well as challenging behaviours including anger/aggression problems and sexual offending. Catani and Sossalla (2015) confirm that the frequency of childhood abuse experiences is high and report that the amount of childhood family abuse predicts PTSD symptom severity in adulthood, suggesting a long-lasting impact of early maltreatment on the mental health in people with intellectual disabilities.

As clinicians, we come across many adults who have become very anxious about what other people think of them because they have experienced frequent name calling, bullying and ridicule because of visible differences and/or an inability to conform with the rules, customs or standards demanded by other people. They may become concerned about being seen to be 'stupid' and their concerns may develop into disabling coping strategies such as withdrawal from social life and new or challenging situations, paranoid ideation and preemptive aggression.

> Interviewer Do you think that people with learning disabilities are more likely to have mental health problems?
> Service user I do, personally.
> Interviewer You do? Why?
> Service user Because I think a lot of ... a lot of the time we've had stigma against disabilities. Throughout our lives. You know? I know I have. I've had people tell me how thick and stupid I am and what have you.
> And it makes it ... it makes it worse, and it makes you believe it. And what have you. And I think that sometimes causes the mental health.
> (http://www.fpld.org.uk/content/assets/pdf/publications/iapt-and-learning-disabilities-report.PDF)

There is also evidence that low IQ increases vulnerability to long-term mental health problems following traumatic experiences (e.g. Murphy and Razza 1998), which may further contribute to the higher rates of mental illness observed in people with intellectual disabilities.

Added to this, people with intellectual disabilities are also more likely to be exposed to social factors that are thought to have a negative impact on (general but also mental) health, in particular poverty, poor housing, unemployment, social exclusion and overt discrimination, all of which are experiences that have been found to cause depression and anxiety symptoms (Glenn et al. 2003). Social exclusion and isolation play an important role in shaping cognitions and self-perception for people with intellectual disabilities, cognitions that mediate depression and anxiety and, as they are more likely to be socially excluded and isolated, they are also more likely to develop mental health problems.

We want to stress here that there are also many people with intellectual disabilities who do not suffer any or few of these risk factors and are able to live rewarding lives and develop many strengths in the context of safe and supportive environments. Even if they have not benefited from such positive backgrounds, many people with intellectual disabilities have good, reciprocal relationships with others and enjoy fulfilling lives. They may have particular strengths such as being 'psychologically minded' (or emotionally intelligent or literate), patient, loyal, interested in particular activities or subjects, or having a good sense of humour. As mental health clinicians we do not often encounter adults with excellent mental health. But many service users we do meet, despite their mental health problems, possess at least some such positive qualities and recognising these 'protective factors' in people's lives can help us to maintain a constructional approach and tailor therapy to people's strengths and take advantage of supports and opportunities in their environments.

Access to CBT for People with Intellectual Disabilities

It is unfortunate that despite our awareness of the greater mental health needs of people with intellectual disabilities, the development of psychosocial interventions has been slow (Hatton 2002) and pharmacological and behavioural interventions have been until recently the treatment of choice despite the evidence that in the long-term talking therapies and in particular CBT can have good outcomes (see Chap. 2).

Despite a 'mainstreaming agenda' (Joint Commissioning Panel for Mental Health 2013) CBT for people with intellectual disabilities in generic mental health services still seems piecemeal and initiatives are vulnerable to service cuts. This clinical work does not appear to be a priority for UK commissioners and policymakers, who generally do not set local goals regarding access to talking therapies for people with intellectual disabilities. Moreover, as clinicians we are concerned that 'mainstreaming' and hence the reduction of specialist services, although presented as an equality issue, will largely be a cost-saving exercise and to the detriment of our clients.

> - Clearer statements of inclusion in services for people with intellectual disabilities
> - Recording systems that allow for monitoring of people with intellectual disabilities seen
> - Training for therapists to include material on working with people with intellectual disabilities, where possible delivered with the involvement of people with intellectual disabilities
> - Pathways for joint working between mainstream mental health and specialist intellectual disabilities services
> - Clear goals and targets regarding use of mental health services by people with intellectual disabilities specified by commissioners and funded appropriately

The Foundation for People with Learning Disabilities (2014) suggests that access to talking therapies can be promoted in the following ways:

Although in some areas mental health workers do receive training in working with people with intellectual disabilities and are allowed by their managers to take a more flexible approach at a slower pace, access to mental health mainstream services remains largely barred to people with intellectual disabilities. Disability (including intellectual disabilities) as a patient characteristic marker rarely features in equality monitoring exercises (e.g. Buffin et al. 2009), which currently makes it impossible to monitor the accessibility of a service.

Access to CBT in specialist services is also hampered by a lack of knowledge, inaccurate and unhelpful attitudes and beliefs amongst potential referrers (e.g. Rossiter and Holmes 2013). Further barriers are created by a lack of confidence, time and resources amongst clinicians, as well as 'diagnostic overshadowing' (e.g. Stenfert Kroese et al. 2001). The latter results in mental health problems (that could be successfully addressed by CBT) not being recognised, as the presenting problems are assumed to be caused by the person's intellectual disabilities.

Within specialist intellectual disabilities services, we find the reverse picture: a wealth of knowledge and expertise in intellectual disabilities yet staff often lack confidence in working with people with mental health problems. The majority of professional and support staff working in intellectual disabilities services come in regular contact with service users who have mental health problems but only a minority receive any training in this complex area (Rose et al. 2007). This means that support workers often feel ill-equipped when they are asked to work with people with mental health problems. Recent evidence indicates that even brief training can increase confidence and improve attitudes and working practices in staff (Costello et al. 2007). Considering that almost half of service users with intellectual disabilities are said have significant mental health problems (see above), such training seems to us to be an essential component of a good-quality service for adults with intellectual disabilities. Staff themselves are very aware of this:

> because of the high level of mental health problems amongst our [service users] … it should be part of the mandatory training and it's a shock to hear, even amongst my esteemed [ID] colleagues, how little they think they've had in terms of mental health training. (member of community team)

> I've been banging on to my line manager for five years, in my supervision and appraisals: I want mental health training, I really want it! I feel this is what's lacking, this is what I feel I'd benefit from most. (member of residential staff team) (Stenfert Kroese et al. 2013)

Mental health service delivery models for people with intellectual disabilities and mental health problems vary across different countries with different positions on the 'specialist intellectual disabilities services-mainstream mental health continuum' but in most Western countries there now appears to be consensus on some form of intellectual disabilities service specialisation (including community outreach and in-patient facilities), strong links and close collaboration between intellectual disabilities specialist and mainstream mental health services, close collaboration between health and social care sectors, and that specialist training needs to be provided for intellectual disabilities and mental health staff to cater for this small but complex group of service users (Cain et al. 2010).

CBT Demand Characteristics

As we described in Chap. 1, CBT is a collaborative, active, directive, time-limited and goal-oriented approach, which gives it a structured, focused form. The term 'collaborative empiricism' has been used to describe the way the therapist and client work together to construct an individual, testable formulation of the problem and the chosen treatment is based on this formulation. It uses a scientific approach to identify, reality test and correct distorted cognitions to bring about long-term change in emotional states (Beck et al. 1979). To do this, clients are asked to identify their negative automatic thoughts (NATs) and keep a thought diary. This facilitates a *metacognitive shift*—the ability to perceive thoughts as opinions rather than statements of fact—so that the process of reality testing can take place. Techniques for reality testing dysfunctional thoughts and assumptions can be practised in sessions guided by the therapist, examining evidence for and against, exploring the usefulness of certain beliefs and developing alternative ways of thinking, perhaps using role play or other activity-based exercises. The client is encouraged to apply these techniques between sessions, using thought diaries and carrying out behavioural experiments to test (and hopefully disprove) assumptions that may be based on dysfunctional thinking. At some point, usually after an initial assessment period, the therapist and the client develop a 'formulation' that explains where the dysfunctional thoughts came from, what they are, what triggers them and what maintains them.

This therapeutic approach, modelled on how scientists gather evidence to prove or disprove their theories, is complex because it uses abstract concepts and processes, and demands a number of intellectual skills and abilities such as:

- conversation skills including language comprehension and expression, turn taking, listening and attending, staying on topic, self-reporting of internal states and cognitions
- identifying thoughts, emotions and behaviours (and distinguishing between them)
- record keeping
- evaluating usefulness of thought patterns and behaviours
- applying techniques such as behavioural experiments
- drawing conclusions from the records and the findings
- contributing to and/or understanding the formulation
- applying coping techniques resulting from the formulation
- maintaining these techniques after the therapy has been completed

Reading through such a list is particularly daunting for therapists who are considering introducing CBT to clients with limited language comprehension and expression, clients who are unlikely to have much experience of two-way conversations where you are expected to take turns and carefully listen and then respond to each other. We found though, in a study using interactional analysis of the patterns of interaction during therapeutic sessions that whilst the therapists asked most of the questions, the clients were able to contribute to the flow of the conversation and play an active part in the dialogues (Jahoda et al. 2009). But to achieve this, the therapist needs to be skilled at encouraging and guiding the client and must be aware of the barriers that stand in the way of creating an equal power balance that allows the client to feel part of the therapeutic process. The techniques that can be used to achieve such therapeutic interactions will be described and discussed in detail in later chapters.

A CBT approach also requires on the part of the client an interest in and motivation to engage and stay engaged in 'psychological thinking' and all the activities that go with it, not just the task demands in the sessions but also the 'homework' and the efforts required to attend the sessions such as getting out of bed in time and arranging (or making sure other people will arrange) transport. The works of Edward Zigler (e.g. Zigler and Hodapp 1986) tell an important developmental story about how people's early experiences can lead to a reduced expectancy of success, a greater reliance on others and a lack of motivation to do things for themselves. He observed that children with intellectual disabilities who had experienced high levels of social deprivation were most prone to become 'verbally dependent and ... wary' (p. 12) in later life and that their ability to perform tasks independently was impaired by

> their high expectancy of failure. This expectancy has been viewed as a consequence of a history of frequent confrontations with tasks which [people with intellectual disabilities] are ill equipped to deal. (p. 15)

So the frequent and painful experiences of failing at tasks where others succeed, so often experienced by people with intellectual disabilities, result not only in increased vulnerability to mental health problems (as we described above) but also in higher levels of dependency and lower levels of motivation to attempt new tasks and take on new challenges. When he observed a 'passive, resigned orientation' in children with intellectual disabilities, Zigler used the term 'learned helplessness' (p. 29), a term introduced by Seligman (1972), to describe their behaviour and to explain how clinical depression may result from perceived or actual lack of control over the outcome of a situation. The theory of learned helplessness emphasises the impact that the environment, especially the environment in the early years of development, can have on functioning in later life. Of course, how a person's learning history affects their emotional and motivational state is the 'bread and butter' of CBT and makes us confident that this approach can be of real benefit for people with intellectual disabilities, as they often report early experiences that have many of the ingredients likely to produce psychological distress in later life.

Whitman (1990) introduced the concept of self-regulation in intellectual disabilities studies. Self-regulation is the term used to describe the ability to manage your own behaviour to achieve goals (Bandura 1986). It has a central place in learning and affects many aspects of life. It incorporates behavioural, cognitive and motivational components (Kendall 1990) and is a significant developmental achievement that gradually 'matures' throughout childhood, adolescence and early adulthood. There are many descriptions of self-regulation in the literature but most agree that it includes setting goals, using appropriate strategies to meet those goals, and monitoring and evaluating your own performance. This requires decision-making, motivation, self-observation and some judgement about the competence of your own performance (Bandura 1991). In short, self-regulation requires a consciousness of self, the belief that the self is an active agent, and an understanding of your own capabilities.

Whitman put forward the hypothesis that for people with intellectual disabilities being able to *apply* what they have learned is more problematic than the learning itself. That is, people with intellectual disabilities can learn many tasks provided they are supported to do so in an appropriate, person-centred way. It is not the learning process that is problematic and impairs their daily functioning, but the application of what is learned, the ability to discriminate between situations when a skill can be effectively applied (e.g. when to cross the road), to judge when to start and when to stop an activity (as in taking a shower or shaking someone's hand) and to appraise past 'performance' and learn from past experiences.

Although these presentations may well have different causes, the concept of executive functioning (Alvarez and Emory 2006) overlaps with Whitman's concept of self-regulation, Zigler's concept of dependency as well as Seligman's concept of learned helplessness. Executive functioning, a neuropsychological term, is rarely mentioned in the context of intellectual disabilities although it seems to us to provide a very useful framework to assess people's ability to function in the therapeutic setting as well as in their daily lives. Executive functioning is a wider concept than self-regulation and refers to the regulation and control of cognitive processes including remembering, reasoning and problem solving as well as planning and executing tasks and routines. As with self-regulation, we find that executive functioning is often deficient in adults with intellectual disabilities. That is, people function reasonably well when they receive frequent and ongoing support in decision-making, long-term planning and implementing and adhering to regular routines but without encouragement, prompting, support and monitoring of others they may flounder. Whether due to a specific learning history or due to 'hard-wired' neurological problems, deficits in executive functioning have important implications for CBT outcome as there is a massive step between learning alternative ways of coping with problems in the therapy room and actually applying these newly learned skills in real life and in time to come.

So far, we have touched on some of the main deficits that we are likely to come across when working with people with intellectual disabilities—problems with communication skills, problem solving and motivation to try out new things and carry out tasks independently. There are other issues to consider when we are planning to adapt standard CBT techniques and practice for people with intellectual disabilities. They include problems with literacy, emotion recognition, attention and memory.

These will be discussed in later chapters and strategies to 'scaffold' some of these deficits will be described.

Our central thesis is that as therapists we need to be prepared to make appropriate and reasonable adjustments in order to compensate for some of these specific deficits in cognitive functioning so that what we ask of people is within the limits of their capability. This will be a central topic in the remaining chapters of this book. After presenting the reader with such a long list of seemingly daunting challenges we are keen to share some of the ways in which we have been able to work successfully with people with intellectual disabilities. We also want to stress that there are a number of benefits to choosing to work according to CBT principles with adults with intellectual disabilities. In our experience, most people with intellectual disabilities appreciate the collaborative client-therapist relationship that is fostered and the directive approach that is so typical of CBT, especially the activity-based tasks, accessible materials and developing a shared formulation.

Recent qualitative studies of clients' with intellectual disabilities experiences and recall of group (MacMahon et al. 2015) and individual therapy (Pert et al. 2013) sessions indicate that when remembering their experiences of CBT therapy most participants focused on social and process issues rather than specific CBT intervention models or techniques applied.

> Participants valued the opportunity to talk about problems with their therapist and benefitted from therapeutic relationships characterised by warmth, empathy and validation. (Pert et al. 2013)

Participants especially appreciated opportunities to develop their relationships with the therapists and (in the case of group therapy) other group members. They also reported their appreciation of opportunities to talk and be listened to and to be treated as an equal and an adult, indicating that the therapeutic alliance (Bordin 1994) and the relationship established is an important component of therapeutic change in CBT interventions for adults with ID.

I felt like an actual person who had the right to tell someone how he feels and not feel daft, because when I used to talk to certain ladies at my place before, when I talked to them they were just sitting there like they weren't listening, because they'd turn their faces and I'd think, 'okay, you're not listening'! (Stenfert Kroese et al. 2016)

How Can We Make CBT Accessible for People with Intellectual Disabilities?

Recent Research Findings on Clients' Cognitive Capacity

McGillivray and Kershaw (2015) compared the effectiveness of CBT, cognitive and behavioural strategies in treating depressive symptoms and NATs of people with mild intellectual disabilities. The results indicate long-term superiority of CBT, with behavioural strategies producing less enduring effects. Group therapy programmes such as 'I'm in Control' (Willner et al. 2013) for people with mild intellectual disabilities and mental health problems tend to focus on teaching participants behavioural coping strategies, and their effectiveness may be further improved if greater emphasis is given to cognitive strategies. But it is important to remember that people with intellectual disabilities are likely to have difficulty understanding the cognitive components of CBT (Dagnan et al. 2009) even if the therapeutic techniques have been adjusted to meet their needs by using simple language and visual aids, involvement of carers and other adaptations.

Although the majority of adults with mild intellectual disabilities appear to be able to link specific events and emotional consequences, they have difficulties in discriminating between thoughts, feelings and behaviours and in understanding cognitive mediation. As already described in Chap. 2, cognitive mediation is the process by which people's thoughts and beliefs determine the impact of a 'neutral' event on their emotional and behavioural responses. Not surprisingly, Dagnan and Chadwick's (1997; Dagnan et al. 2000) research suggests that people with ID find it more difficult to identify an appropriate mediating cognition when there is incongruence between the given event and the emotion (e.g. some friends do not say 'hello' and you feel happy) compared to when the emotion matches the event. Chapter 4 will describe how cognitive mediation can be assessed and used in therapy sessions.

People who lack some of these prerequisite skills for CBT can benefit from a pre-therapy structured intervention to teach them CBT's core concepts such as cognitive mediation (e.g. Sams et al. 2006). Two studies have so far examined whether preparatory training can enhance the cognitive skills of people with mild to moderate intellectual disabilities (Bruce et al. 2010; Vereenooghe et al. 2013).

Bruce et al. (2010) found that adults with intellectual disabilities who received structured training in CBT skills were better at creating links between thoughts and feelings compared to a control group but training had no effect on participants' ability to discriminate feelings, thoughts and behaviours. This may be related to the nature of the discrimination task, which asks people to identify whether a number of words and phrases represent something they 'think', 'feel' or 'do'. In our experience people can become particularly confused when they lack personal experience with some task items, which tells us that we should use individually tailored and personally meaningful assessment instruments whenever possible rather than relying on measures that demand too much abstract thinking of our clients. Another problem concerns the way that some task items are worded, such as 'I don't know what to do for the best'. The use of the word 'do' may mislead some people, 'forcing' them to respond that this is a behaviour rather than a thought. On the other hand, when asked whether 'upset' is a thought, emotion or behaviour, one of our service users answered that 'upset' is something he does (i.e. a behaviour) because 'I do. I *do* get very upset.' We also find that in therapeutic conversations some people will use the word 'feel' as synonymous to 'think'. This is reflected in the response of someone who was asked to say whether 'I don't know what to do for the best' was 'something you think, feel or do' answered, 'Feel, I *feel* I don't know what to do for the best.'

Vereenooghe and colleagues (2015) investigated the impact of computerised training on people's cognitive mediation skills, measured by tasks developed by Dagnan and colleagues. Their results indicate that the intervention was effective in increasing participants' ability to choose the appropriate feeling when they were given congruent pairings of events and thoughts, but had no effect on their ability to identify the correct mediating cognition when provided with either congruent or incongruent pairings of events and emotions.

In our clinical experience people with intellectual disabilities are better at correctly identifying feelings compared to thoughts and behaviours. This was also the finding of Hebblethwaite et al. (2011) who observed that although people with intellectual disabilities and people with normal cognitive function were equally able to identify and describe their feelings about an emotional real-life experience, those with intellectual disabilities were less able to talk about their inferential beliefs.

Other Factors: Meeting Halfway?

Although we think that these prerequisite skills are important, we argue that the evaluation of clients' capacity for participating in and benefiting from CBT should not only depend on their performance on formal assessments of CBT skills. There are a number of other critical factors that influence the successful implementation of CBT in people with ID such as the quality of the therapeutic relationship, motivation to participate in therapy, psychological thinking and self-efficacy and the engagement of carers in treatment and the support they give.

Also, we need to consider how we can cater for people for whom spoken and written language is problematic. Clements (1997) emphasises how narrow our focus can be when he draws our attention to the various modalities that people can employ to make sense of the world—auditory, visual, olfactory, tactile, kinaesthetic. He points out that people with and without disabilities vary in what they attend to and how they experience the outside world. CBT's focus on higher order levels of verbal analysis neglects other ways of experiencing and representing the world and in which information can be processed, beliefs are formed and skills are learned.

> There is no doubt that the cognitive functioning of human beings is dazzlingly diverse and correspondingly complex. (p. 163)

As CBT therapists we do not have to limit ourselves to verbal communication but should explore the use of visual media—pictures, photos, cartoons, film, facial expressions and posture—as well as modelling, movement and signing in order to communicate with our clients, help them understand, learn and remember and prompt them to apply some of the alternative ways of coping with their problems. Such adaptations have been found to have good results for other client groups such as children, older adults and people with traumatic brain injury.

We do not consider it realistic (and certainly would not advise) that CBT therapists demand or expect that all 'necessary' skills as listed above are learned by their clients before therapy commences. Our goal must not (and cannot) be *remediation* of all cognitive deficits. Instead, we recommend that when after assessment and a certain amount of psychoeducational input, a *compensation* approach is an acceptable and desirable option, finding a way round the functional difficulty that may be different from the 'normal' way but can achieve the same outcome. This is analogous to ensuring a person has a good mobility aid after physiotherapy assessment has indicated that learning how to walk is not a realistic option. This has implications for us as therapists who, instead of denying access to therapy because of deficits or alternatively insisting that clients need to learn prerequisite skills (such as being able to distinguish between thoughts, emotions and behaviour before therapy can begin), have to change our methods to compensate for their particular deficits.

With regard to therapists adopting a flexible, person-centred approach to CBT, Whittington and Grey (2014) make a distinction between metacompetence and unfocused practice. The term 'metacompetence' was introduced into the therapeutic literature by Roth and Pilling (2007) and can be defined as a therapist's higher order competences that focus on the ability to implement models in a way that is flexible and tailored to the needs of the client. There are generic metacompetencies such as the capacity to use clinical judgement when implementing treatment models and adapt interventions in response to client feedback and, for example, to be able to judge when it is appropriate to use and respond to humour. CBT-specific competencies include the ability to formulate and apply CBT models to each individual client and select and apply the most appropriate intervention, as well as being able to structure sessions, adopt the right pace and manage any unforeseen obstacles. In the case of clients with intellectual disabilities, the last three competencies are particularly relevant as the therapist must be skilled in working with people whose comprehension, attention span and ability to take part in a conversation between equal partners may all be deficient in some way. Whittington and Grey talk of *artful delivery* and advocate that there is a delicate balance between the 'science of CBT and its artful delivery': on the one hand there is a risk of being overly rigid in an attempt to adhere to the protocol and on the other hand there is a risk of drifting away from effective methods in the belief you are helpfully flexible. The concept of *metacompetent adherence* gives a framework to bridge that gap. The advantages and disadvantages of using 'loose' or 'tight' principles and tactics and techniques are outlined in the box below.

	Tactics and technique: tight	Tactics and technique: loose
Principles: tight	**Competent adherence** CBT applied in the standard way as in random clinical trials (RCTs). Suited to learning CBT and to specific problem types with specific protocols. Likely to be effective if there is a good fit between the specific approach and the specific case/problem.	**Metacompetent adherence** Appropriate adaptation of CBT tactics and techniques. Suited for cases that don't fit the usual guidelines. Different to therapist 'drift' as adaptation is theory and evidence based. More likely to be needed with complex cases and easier with greater clinical experience.
Principles: loose	**Rigid practice** CBT applied rigidly without recourse to principles—just thinking about what to do next without properly basing this on a formulation. Can be aversive for clients and have a negative impact on outcome.	**Unfocused practice** Unfocused tactics and erratic use of technique without recourse to CBT principles. This is the culmination of therapist 'drift'—like 'having a chat'. Does not resemble CBT and likely to be less effective.

Taken from Whittington and Grey (2014)

A further metacompetence that in our experience is essential for applying CBT successfully for people with intellectual disabilities is adopting a *situational competence* or *distributed competence* (Booth and Booth 1998) perspective. As people with intellectual disabilities are almost always to some extent dependent on other people in their day-to-day life, we must acknowledge and work with the inhibitory or facilitating influence of the environment and in particular the role of other people in determining competence. A common first hurdle encountered by therapists is how to motivate support workers and other carers to enable the client to attend the appointments. Attending CBT sessions is not always perceived to be a priority in the busy working lives of staff and family members and that DNA rates are high in intellectual disabilities services is by no means solely due to clients opting out of treatment. Another challenge for CBT therapists is to help staff or carers recognise the importance of allowing and encouraging clients to use as much self-determination as possible in their lives, and to promote *competence promoting* versus *competence inhibiting* support (Tucker and Johnson 1989). When the carers' input becomes overprotective or, on the other hand, when they expect too much of the client too soon, the therapeutic outcome is unlikely to be good. These issues will be discussed in more detail in Chap. 10.

> **Key Points**
> - There is a high prevalence of mental health problems amongst adults with intellectual disability.
> - Access to mental health services, especially talking therapies, remains problematic for our clients.
> - Access to CBT services is hampered by a lack of knowledge and confidence amongst generic therapists.
> - Staff in learning disability services report that they lack training in mental health issues.

- Although the demand characteristics of CBT appear many and complex, a skilled therapist can adapt the methods and materials to make it accessible to people with intellectual disabilities.
- Learned helplessness, self-regulation and executive functioning are related and relevant concepts that must be considered in the context of the potential of CBT to have long-lasting benefits for our clients.
- Instead of a remediation approach to facilitating access to CBT, we must consider a compensation approach.
- When adapting CBT practice for our clients, we must avoid 'drifting' into unfocused ways of working. Instead, we should aim for 'metacompetent adherence' to the CBT model.

References

Alvarez, J. A., & Emory, E. (2006). Executive function and the frontal lobes: A meta-analytic review. *Neuropsychology Review, 16*(1), 17–42.

Bandura, A. (1986). The explanatory and predictive scope of self-efficacy theory. *Journal of Clinical and Social Psychology, 4*, 359–373.

Bandura, A. (1991). Social cognitive theory of self-regulation. *Organizational Behavior and Human Decision Processes, 50*, 248–287.

Beck, A. T., Rush, A., Shaw, B., & Emery, G. (1979). *Cognitive therapy for depression*. New York: Wiley.

Booth, T., & Booth, W. (1998). *Growing up with parents who have learning difficulties*. London: Routledge.

Bordin, E. (1994). Theory and research on the therapeutic working alliance: New directions. In A. Horvath & L. Greenberg (Eds.), *The working alliance: Theory, research and practice* (pp. 13–37). New York: Wiley.

Bruce, M., Collins, S., Langdon, P., Powlitch, S., & Reynolds, S. (2010). Does training improve understanding of core concepts in cognitive behaviour therapy by people with intellectual disabilities? A randomised experiment. *British Journal of Clinical Psychology, 49*, 1–13.

Buffin, J., Ahmed, N., & Singh, M. (2009). Using a community engagement approach to ensure equality of access, experience and outcome from the IAPT programme in the North West of England. Report UCLAN/NHS North West.

Cain, N. N., Davidson, P. W., Dosen, A., et al. (2010). An international perspective of mental health services for people with intellectual disability. In N. Bouras & G. Holt (Eds.), *Mental health services for adults with intellectual disability: Strategies and solutions.* London: Psychology Press.

Catani, C., & Sossalla, I. M. (2015). Child abuse predicts adult PTSD symptoms among individuals diagnosed with intellectual disabilities. *Frontiers in Psychology, 6,* 1600. Published online 2015 Oct 19 doi: 10.3389/fpsyg.2015.01600.

Clements, J. (1997). Sustaining a cognitive psychology for people with learning disabilities. In B. Stenfert Kroese, D. Dagnan, & K. Loumidis (Eds.), *Cognitive-behavioural therapy for people with learning disabilities* (pp. 162–181). London: Routledge.

Cooper, S. A., Smiley, E., Morrison, J., Williamson, A., & Allan, L. (2007). An epidemiological investigation of affective disorders with a population-based cohort of 1023 adults with intellectual disabilities. *Psychological Medicine, 37,* 873–882.

Costello, H., Bouras, N., & Davies, H. (2007). The role of training in improving community care staff awareness of mental health problems in people with intellectual disabilities. *Journal of Applied Research in Intellectual Disabilities, 20*(3), 228–235.

Dagnan, D., & Chadwick, P. (1997). Cognitive-behaviour therapy for people with learning disabilities: Assessment and intervention. In B. Stenfert Kroese, D. Dagnan, & K. Loumidis (Eds.), *Cognitive-behaviour therapy for people with learning disabilities* (pp. 110–123). London: Routledge.

Dagnan, D., Chadwick, P., & Proudlove, J. (2000). Toward an assessment of suitability of people with mental retardation for cognitive therapy. *Cognitive Therapy and Research, 24,* 627–636.

Dagnan, D., Mellor, K., & Jefferson, C. (2009). Assessment of cognitive therapy skills for people with intellectual disability. *Advances in Mental Health and Learning Disabilities, 3,* 25–30.

Department of Health. (2011). Talking therapies: A four year plan. www.iapt.nhs.uk

Foundation for People with Learning Disabilities. (2014). Feeling down – Improving the mental health of people with learning disabilities. http://www.learningdisabilities.org.uk/content/assets/pdf/publications/feeling-down-report-2014.pdf

Glenn, E., Bihm, E. M., & Lammers, W. J. (2003). Depression, anxiety and relevant cognitions in persons with mental retardation. *Journal of Autism and Developmental Disorders, 33*(1), 69–76.

Hatton, C. (2002). Psychosocial interventions for adults with intellectual disabilities and mental health problems: A review. *Journal of Mental Health, 11*(4), 357–374.

Hebblethwaite, A., Jahoda, A., & Dagnan, D. (2011). Talking about real-life events: An investigation into the ability of people with intellectual disabilities to make links between their beliefs and emotions within dialogue. *Journal of Applied Research in Intellectual Disabilities, 24*(6), 543–553.

Jahoda, A., Dagnan, D., Stenfert Kroese, B., Pert, C., & Trower, P. (2009). Cognitive behavioural therapy: From face to face interaction to a broader contextual understanding of change. *Journal of Intellectual Disability Research, 53*(9), 759–771.

Joint Commissioning Panel for Mental Health. (2013). Guidance for commissioning public mental health services. http://www.jcpmh.info/resource/guidance-for-commissioning-public-mental-health-services/

Kendall, P. C. (1990). Challenges for cognitive strategy training: The case of mental retardation. *American Journal on Mental Retardation, 94*, 365–367.

Lindsay, W. R., Steele, L., Smith, A. H., Quinn, K., & Allan, R. (2006). A community forensic intellectual disability service: Twelve year follow up of referrals, analysis of referral patterns and assessment of harm reduction. *Legal and Criminological Psychology, 11*(1), 113–130.

McGillivray, J., & Kershaw, M. (2015). Do we need both cognitive and behavioural components in interventions for depressed mood in people with mild intellectual disability? *Journal of Intellectual Disability Research, 59*(2), 105–115.

MacMahon, P., Stenfert Kroese, B., Jahoda, A., Stimpson, A., Rose, N., Rose, J., Townson, J., Hood, K., & Willner, P. (2015). 'It's made all of us bond since that course…' – A qualitative study of service users' experiences of a CBT anger management group intervention. *Journal of Intellectual Disability Research, 59*(4), 342–352.

Morgan, V. A., Leonard, H., Bourke, J., & Jablensky, A. (2008). Intellectual disability co-occurring with schizophrenia and other psychiatric illness: Population-based study. *British Journal of Psychiatry, 193*, 364–372.

Murphy, L., & Razza, N. (1998). Domestic violence against women with mental retardation. In A. Roberts (Ed.), *Battered women and their families* (pp. 271–290). New York: Springer.

Pert, C., Jahoda, A., Stenfert Kroese, B., Trower, P., Dagnan, D., & Selkirk, M. (2013). Cognitive behavioural therapy from the perspective of clients with mild intellectual disabilities: A qualitative investigation of process issues. *Journal of Intellectual Disability Research, 57*(4), 359–369.

Rose, N., O'Brien, A., & Rose, J. (2007). Investigating staff knowledge and attitudes towards working with adults with learning disabilities and mental health difficulties. *Advances in Mental Health and Learning Disabilities, 1*(3), 52–59.

Rossiter, R., & Holmes, S. (2013). Access all areas: Creative adaptations for CBT with people with cognitive impairments – Illustrations and issues. *The Cognitive Behaviour Therapist, 6*(4). doi:10.1017/S1754470X13000135.

Roth, A. D., & Pilling, S. (2007). *The competences required to deliver effective cognitive and behavioural therapy for people with depression and with anxiety disorders*. London: Department of Health.

Sams, K., Collins, S., & Reynolds, S. (2006). Cognitive therapy abilities in people with learning disabilities. *Journal of Applied Research in Intellectual Disabilities, 19*, 25–33.

Seligman, M. E. P. (1972). Learned helplessness. *Annual Review of Medicine., 23*(1), 407–412. doi:10.1146/annurev.me.23.020172.002203.

Stenfert Kroese, B., Dewhurst, D., & Holmes, G. (2001). Diagnosis and drugs: Help or hindrance when people with learning disabilities have psychological problems? *British Journal of Learning Disabilities, 29*(1), 26–33.

Stenfert Kroese, B., Rose, J., Heer, K., & O'Brien, A. (2013). Mental health services for adults with intellectual disabilities – What do service users and staff think of them? *Journal of Applied Research in Intellectual Disabilities, 26*(1), 3–13.

Stenfert Kroese, B., Willott, S., Taylor, F., Smith, P., Graham, R., Rutter, T., Stott, A., & Willner, P. (2016). Trauma-focussed cognitive-behaviour therapy for people with mild intellectual disabilities: Outcomes of a pilot study. *Advances in Mental Health and Intellectual Disabilities, 10*(5), 299–310.

Tucker, B. M., & Johnson, O. (1989). Competence promoting vs. competence inhibiting social support for mentally retarded mothers. *Human Organization, 48*, 95–107.

Vereenooghe, L., & Langdon, P. E. (2013). Psychological therapies for people with intellectual disabilities: A systematic review and meta-analysis. *Research in Developmental Disabilities, 34*(11), 4085–4102.

Vereenooghe, L., Reynolds, S., Gega, L., & Langdon, P. E. (2015). Can a computerised training paradigm assist people with intellectual disabilities to learn cognitive mediation skills? A randomised experiment. *Behaviour Research and Therapy, 71*, 10–19.

Whitman, T. L. (1990). Self-regulation and mental retardation. *American Journal on Mental Retardation, 94*(4), 347–362.

Whittington, A., & Grey, N. (2014). *How to become a more effective CBT therapist -mastering metacompetence in clinical practice*. Oxford: Wiley Blackwell.

Willner, P., Rose, J., Jahoda, A., Stenfert Kroese, B., Felce, D., Cohen, D., MacMahon, P., Stimpson, A., Rose, N., Gillespie, D., Shead, J., Lammie, C., Woodgate, C., Townson, J., Nuttall, J., & Hood, K. (2013). Group-based cognitive-behavioural anger management for people with mild to moderate intellectual disabilities: Cluster randomised controlled trial. *The British Journal of Psychiatry, 203*(4), 288–296.

Zigler, E., & Hodapp, R. (1986). *Understanding mental retardation*. New York: Cambridge University Press.

4

Assessment and Setting the Scene for Cognitive Behaviour Therapy

Rather than presenting a truncated CBT manual, the aim of this chapter and Chap. 5 will be to flesh out the therapist's role when delivering therapy, highlighting key decisions the therapist has to make (therapy process) and describing the nature of the intervention itself (therapy content). Whilst it is hoped that these steps offer a guide, these are not meant to be prescriptive. Instead, it is hoped that the account given will equip the therapist with the 'know-how' to deal with some of the main challenges they will encounter when using CBT with clients who have an intellectual disability. Given the widely different needs and abilities of people with intellectual disabilities, we don't expect that the suggestions made here will be relevant in every case.

Making a Start

As discussed in previous chapters, the first stage of therapy concerns establishing rapport with clients, obtaining a history and finding out about their current circumstances. A good understanding of the CBT model is important, because whilst many therapeutic tasks are described separately in this chapter for the purpose of clarity, in fact they are often overlapping and interlinked. For example, showing a genuine interest in the person's life and trying to understand their thoughts and feelings as part of an initial assessment should also help to build rapport and can act as an important catalyst to change.

At the first session, the therapist should check out what the client knows about the referral, what their feelings are about coming to the session, their view of their problems and what they want help with. Establishing shared goals for therapy will help to instil hope and increase motivation. Care needs to be taken with the pace of the sessions, ensuring that clients grasp what is happening and why. It can be challenging at the beginning of therapy to create structure and a sense of direction, whilst at the same time adapting the approach to the particular needs of the individual. In some instances, where people have speech difficulties or an idiosyncratic way of expressing themselves, it may take a little time for the therapist to tune into what the client is saying. The reason for pacing sessions differently for people with intellectual disabilities is not simply because they are slower to achieve change but also because the therapist needs to ensure he or she is making the appropriate adaptations.

The onus at the start of therapy is not just for the therapist to get to know the client, it is also for the client to get to know the therapist and to begin to develop an understanding of what is to be covered in sessions. Going to a first appointment with any health professional can be anxiety provoking. The expectations and emotions someone brings to meeting a therapist for the first time might be linked to their understanding of what will happen, their optimism for change and perhaps whether they feel in control of the process or rather helpless. In fact, people's positive expectations and hopes for therapy have been shown to be associated with more successful outcomes (Delsignore and Schnyder 2007). There may be a number of reasons why this is the case. For example, being more optimistic about the possibility of change might make it more likely that people will engage wholeheartedly in the therapeutic process. Amy Kilbane proposed a model of therapy expectations and motivation in adults with an intellectual disability, which is shown below (Kilbane and Jahoda 2011).

Making a Start 57

Therapy Expectations and Motivatons

Conceptual Model

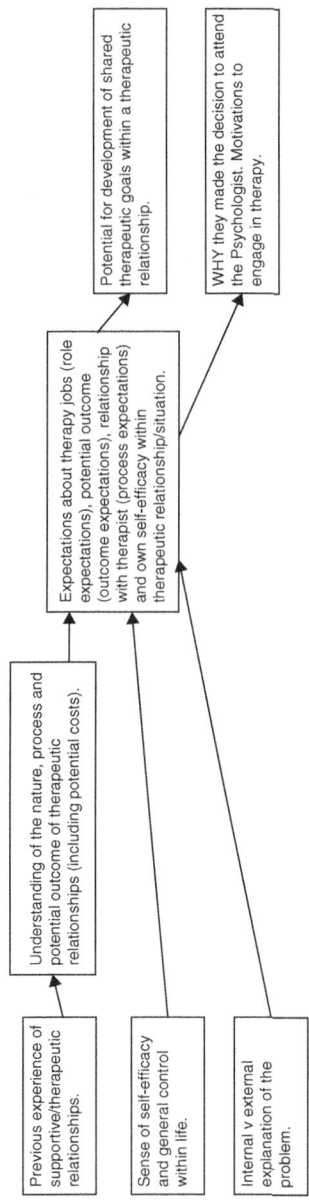

One of the main points to be taken from this model is that a person's expectations about engaging with any psychological therapy, including CBT, need to be understood in the context of their current and previous experience of helping relationships. Feeling that they are making a choice to meet with the therapist might also have a bearing on their motivation to engage with therapy. In our own clinical practice, we have found that concerns clients with intellectual disabilities have about attending therapy are very often related to issues of choice and autonomy. For example, many clients are unsure of their right to refuse therapy and may meet with a CBT therapist for the first time without having been asked whether they want psychological help. Others might lack awareness of the rules of confidentiality in therapy, causing them to worry that information they discuss will be passed on to others.

For some clients, their early apprehensiveness may simply stem from a lack of familiarity with the circumstances that surround therapy. Others will have had extensive input from health care and social care professionals and may expect that CBT will follow a similar pattern, either to good or to bad effect. In order to overcome other misconceptions and avoid barriers to engagement, the therapist should make it clear, ideally before the first appointment, that therapy is optional and that the client can stop attending at any stage. To help uncover fears or identify areas of confusion, at the outset it can help to directly ask the client whether they had any worries about coming to the appointment. This can have the dual benefit of uncovering fears and reassuring the client that their views are central to the process of therapy and will be taken seriously. In our experience, many clients can benefit from access to leaflets or DVDs about therapy before therapy begins (Dunn et al. 2006). If similar materials are not available to the therapist he or she should make a point of discussing choice, confidentiality and the involvement of carers during the first session. Talking through the following checklist information can help to address common misconceptions.

> **What Does Therapy Involve?**
> - When we meet we will talk about problems you want help with.
> - We will work together to try to find new ways of dealing with your problem.
> - I will not give you medication.
> - I will not pass information to others except if you or someone else might come to some harm. I will always tell you.
> - Therapy will not last forever. We will stop meeting when you feel better or if it is not helping you.

In a study where we asked individuals with intellectual disabilities about their experience of CBT (Pert et al. 2013), most participants told us that even though they felt the therapy had been helpful they did not necessarily expect the benefits to last when therapy finished. It seemed that what they expected (or wanted) was a long-term supportive relationship rather than a time-limited intervention. Bearing this in mind, the therapist may feel it is especially important to make the time-limited nature of the intervention clear. However, some clients' wish for a longer term confiding relationship is quite understandable, especially when they don't have other confiding relationships in their lives. Involving significant others in the therapeutic process might be one way of helping to ensure continuing support. Another option is to offer follow-up sessions, perhaps a month apart, to help clients maintain progress. Whilst in some quarters this may seem inefficient and a waste of limited resources, using a 'light touch' to support clients to cope with continuing difficulties, or new problems that arise, before they become major issues helps to avoid further referrals and offers a sense of ongoing support for clients who need to build confidence in their ability to use strategies.

Another point to take account of at this early stage of therapy is the role of significant others in the client's life. In most cases, the person will arrive at the first session accompanied by a family member or worker. Understandably, the client will often ask if the support person can accompany them to meet with the therapist. Far from being problematic, this can be reassuring for some clients. The support person may be able to assist the client to tell their story or fill in gaps that the client cannot recall in detail. Sometimes a client may have an idiosyncratic way of speaking or fail to mention key details about their lives and the support person can make useful interventions. There are also some occasions when the support person can help the therapist to pitch questions at the right level, perhaps breaking down a complicated question the therapist has asked to make it more manageable for the client or putting it in language that is more familiar for them. However, some clients require a family member or a carer to support them to travel to appointments purely for practical reasons, and it doesn't necessarily follow that they wish to be supported within the therapy session. So the therapist needs to find out what the client is comfortable with. Clearly, preferences will vary from individual to individual. Some clients want to have a carer present during the initial session, but wish to be seen on their own thereafter when they grow in confidence. Others may be happy for their family member, or carer, to be involved throughout, or for the therapist to invite input from carers 'as required', perhaps for homework tasks, keeping diaries and monitoring systems.

The other point to bear in mind is that it may not always be straightforward for the client to state that they want to see the therapist on their own, either because they are worried about upsetting their supporter or because the supporter is too dominant. One way of dealing with this is to suggest having a little time on your own with clients at the end of one of the first sessions, to check out what they want to do.

Before We Start: Where to Meet?

A point to consider that rarely arises when working with other populations is where to meet with the client. In services in the UK, clinical psychologists often work with people who have intellectual disabilities on an outreach basis, rather than expecting them to attend a clinic. Many individuals may not be able to travel independently to the clinic or lack the support to do so. Others may not have the confidence to make the journey, lead rather chaotic lives or have emotional problems such as agoraphobia that make it difficult for them to attend. However, not everyone agrees that this is a good idea and when writing this book we have discovered that we hold rather different views.

There are undoubtedly pros and cons to working on an outreach basis with clients. Care has to be taken to ensure that a private space is available to meet with the person, particularly if they live with family or in a shared house, where people's privacy is not always respected. It is not a good idea to deliver therapy in a person's bedroom at home or in a living room or in a public room where you can be overheard or there are interruptions from other people. Nor is daytime television a helpful aid to therapy. You also need to be very careful that you are not compromising the person's right to confidentiality by visiting them where they live or work, by drawing attention to the fact that they are receiving help for their mental health problems. So if you are proposing to meet with a client on an outreach basis then be very careful to check that they are happy with this arrangement. When negotiating the role of carers, it is worth noting that some clients with intellectual disabilities may have relatively little opportunity for private conversations and might value the opportunity for individual sessions. One client told us:

> I felt a bit more comfortable one to one, because you can talk about things that are private and confidential. Any, like … eh problems that you've got that you don't want anybody else to know because it's private, you know. (Ref Male, aged 28, referred for anger)

Of course, it is possible to offer privacy and a confiding relationship alongside the sensitive involvement of carers. As noted in Chap. 2, the aim is to foster competence promoting rather than competence inhibiting support.

Another advantage of asking the client to make the effort to travel to a clinic setting is that it sets the tone for sessions, making it clear that therapy is an important and active process and clients have a role to play in working towards change. On the other hand, seeing people on an outreach basis can demonstrate the therapist's commitment to supporting clients to achieve change. Making an effort to reach out to clients also helps to counter health inequalities because those who are socially marginalised and perhaps lead chaotic lives should not have to miss out on therapy.

Meeting with clients where they live can also provide insight into the wider context of a client's life. This insight is important for therapists. CBT is a talking therapy and relies on intersubjectivity or a shared understanding between the therapist and client to maintain a therapeutic dialogue. People with intellectual disabilities sometimes fail to appreciate what the therapist does or does not know about them. If, as a therapist, you do not know the people, places or events that the client is talking about, then it is easy to misunderstand what is being said or you may fail to pick up on salient issues. Finally, working on an outreach basis can provide the therapist with a clearer sense of what might be possible for the person to achieve and the constraints they live under or opportunities they are afforded. Knowing what support a client receives from services and their relationship with support workers or family members can be very useful. Coming into direct contact with significant others in the client's life also makes it more straightforward to involve them in the therapeutic process, if this is agreed to be a helpful approach.

Hearing the Client's Story and Creating a Safe Place

As with any therapy, a good starting point is to invite the client to tell their story in their own words. As well as offering insight into their perspective, distinct from that of the referrer, this process can reveal the person's view of their world, self and others.

These early clinical discussions will also help the therapist to gauge clients' ability to engage in a therapeutic dialogue. Early sessions can offer insight into people's ability to reflect on and describe their experiences, their interpersonal skills and the ability to link their experiences and emotions. In our experience of supervising clinical psychologists in training, one of the main concerns expressed is in relation to client communication difficulties, with fears that these will disrupt the easy flow of therapeutic conversation. Adaptations will depend on the specific nature of the client's communication problems. A good starting point when you don't understand what a client has said is to offer reassurance that you take responsibility to overcome communication problems. The therapist can start with general questions followed by more specific questions to home in on the topic and clarify what has been said. We usually find that clients' idiosyncratic speech soon becomes easier to understand. We urge the therapist to persevere and adapt. Further adaptations will be discussed later in Chap. 7.

Therapeutic work of any hue is built on the foundations of the therapeutic relationship (Gilbert and Leahy 2007). Interestingly, much that is written about adapting CBT for people with intellectual disabilities tends to be focused on therapeutic technique and the skills that people with intellectual disabilities need in order to engage positively with the techniques. In general adult mental health there has been growing interest in the importance of so-called non-specific factors in psychotherapy, such as the therapeutic relationship. Interestingly, when we interviewed participants with intellectual disabilities about their experience of CBT, they highlighted the therapeutic relationship as one of the most helpful aspects of therapy. When people are socially marginalised and disempowered, the therapeutic relationship is likely to be especially salient for them (Pert et al. 2013).

It is well known that the therapeutic bond is strengthened when clients feel listened to, understood, and they view the therapist as an ally (Joyce and Piper 1998). The benefits go beyond rapport building, as good therapeutic relationships are associated with improved treatment outcomes and greater overall client satisfaction with therapy (Bachelor and Horvarth 1999; Beutler et al. 1994). It has been suggested that the supportive nature of the therapeutic relationship may be even more crucial for clients with intellectual disabilities due to a lack of close, confiding relationships in their lives (Pert et al. 2013; McDonald et al. 2003).

> But you can actually see by (therapist) that she's listening, because she's looking straight at you when, when you're talking to her and she just listens as well. (Male, aged 32, referred for anxiety and anger)

Setting the Scene

Setting an agenda is the usual method of introducing structure when beginning CBT work. The manner in which the agenda is agreed with clients with an intellectual disability is important and time should be taken to discuss what will be covered and to negotiate the content. This is a good example of 'learning by doing'. If the client has sufficient literary skills you could ask them to write out the agenda, ensuring that the language used is straightforward and accessible. Otherwise, you could ask the client to take on the task of ticking off agenda points as they are covered in the session. Depending on clients' literacy skills, drawings can be used to represent the different issues to be covered. As discussed previously, giving the clients an active role in the sessions from the start sets the tone for collaborative working. Bill Lindsay, a pioneer in adapting CBT for people with intellectual disabilities (see Lindsay et al. 2015), pointed out that an agenda is particularly useful for clients because it helps to make sessions predictable and scaffolds their involvement. In other words, if you know what to expect in sessions then you are in a better position to make a contribution. The agenda can also be helpful when working with distractible clients.

Finding the Right Pace

The usual process of gathering relevant background information will take longer than usual, so the therapist should be mindful of the pace and timing of questions, especially in the first few assessment sessions. This is particularly important when working with clients who have expressive communication difficulties, as the demands on the client will be heightened. It is vital that the therapist does not sacrifice rapport in order to push ahead with assessment materials. Yet even with a slower pace of questioning most clients with intellectual disabilities are unable to answer routine historical information during assessment, for example, regarding their education, medical history and current health issues. Consequently, the therapist might ask for the client's agreement to gather essential information from carers or other health professionals involved. To maintain rapport and the flow of early sessions, it may be best to begin by focusing mainly on here and now issues, or those that the client views as most pressing, and gather the historical aspects of background history in subsequent sessions when the client has had a greater opportunity to settle into therapy.

In order to understand the impact of the client's disability on their day-to-day lives, it is useful to get a sense of the client's current level of autonomy, dependency on others and current support networks. Perhaps more importantly, the therapist should be vigilant to signs of a mismatch between the client's perception of their need for support and the supports currently in place. In some cases clients may wish more autonomy in their life, whilst others may feel undersupported or abandoned.

Many clients will have received long-standing services from a range of health and social care professionals. For that reason, it is often helpful to draw a visual 'map' of (i) current support networks, for example, family, friends, health and social care professionals, and (ii) their regular activities. As well as acting as a useful memory aid for the therapist, the process of populating this map on a flip chart with the client can reveal the relationships and activities of most importance to clients. Given the key role of support services for many people with an intellectual disability, it is important to consider how support provision might impact on difficulties, or act as a protective factor. Some of the day-to-day challenges that individuals face will relate to their social circumstances and the impacts of having an intellectual disability. Few clients with intellectual disabilities will be in paid employment. Managing finances on limited social benefits is challenging enough, but especially for those who lack numeracy and literacy skills.

As well as possible problems remembering details of what has happened in the past some clients will have difficulty establishing the correct sequence of events. One way to help clients develop their life story is by drawing a timeline, which charts key life events on a continuum from childhood to the present time. It helps to illustrate this with drawings to make the process engaging and aid memory. Again, the timeline chart can then serve as a useful reference point that can be returned to throughout therapy.

Is CBT Suitable?

At this initial assessment phase, the therapist has the additional task of establishing whether the client has the essential skills to engage in talking therapy; such as sufficient communication, memory, attention and emotional understanding. However, there is no available benchmark of the skills required and the therapist will have to use his or her judgement, based on the client's presentation and information available, to decide if they are able to engage in sessions and are likely to benefit from taking part. This will require adequate expressive and receptive verbal ability, and sufficient emotional understanding. Other key indicators are the ability to remain on topic or return to topic when prompted to do so, the ability to reflect on experiences, and the ability to retain necessary information from previous sessions when given the necessary repetition of that information and memory aids. Obviously one of the core skills of the CBT approach is cognitive mediation. This is something we will go on to consider in the next chapter, when we look at the process of socialising clients to the CBT model.

In some cases it may be helpful to verify aspects of clients' emotional and social cognitive understanding by way of direct assessment. The Reed and Clements's assessment of emotional understanding was one of the first self-assessments used for this purpose (Reed and Clements 1989). Otherwise, ad hoc assessments can be incorporated into early therapy sessions, such as exploring the client's ability to distinguish emotions from photographs of facial expression (e.g. Eckman 1993), asking clients to either label each emotion shown ('How is this person feeling?') or choose an identified emotion from options ('Point to the sad face'). DVDs can also be used to explore body language and tone of voice associated with different emotions. These methods offer insights into the clients' ability to detect emotion in others and can then be used as a basis to go on to talk about triggers for the clients' own emotions. Often clients do not identify emotions when first invited to talk about feelings, yet can be helped to do so by showing photographs or video clips of emotion and asking 'When did you feel like this?' and 'What happened to make you feel that way?' This is one example of how the therapist can scaffold the demands of therapy, adapting the process to suit the client's level of ability.

Some clients will require a more graded approach to help them distinguish their emotions. This can be done by using an emotions map or linear chart that chunks emotions according to 'good feelings' (e.g. *happy, excited, calm*) and 'bad feelings' (e.g. *angry, sad, uptight*). The therapist and client can work through emotion cards and categorise these. The next step would be to link emotional triggers to each category (*feel good/feel bad*), then choose an emotion from that category, as shown below.

Therapist: When you fell out with your brother (emotional trigger) did it make you feel good or bad?
Client: I felt bad.
Therapist: I see. Well let's have a look at the Bad Feelings cards (*angry, sad, uptight*). Did you have any of these feelings when you fell out with your brother?
Client: I'd say uptight.
Therapist: Okay, so, when you fell out with your brother you felt uptight.

The use of photographs of each emotion can improve engagement and offer clients non-verbal cues to help them choose the appropriate emotion. As mentioned, the therapist might also use DVDs and extracts from films or popular television shows to explore a range of expressed emotions. One engaging option is the film animation 'Inside Out' which explores the emotions of a young girl, and emphasises the important role of each emotion.

As well as exploring the clients' emotional understanding, gleaning other information regarding their wider socio-cognitive understanding will help the therapist to pitch therapy correctly and identify aspects of the client's cognitive difficulties or thinking style that could impact on the therapy process. Other information to be gathered by the therapist during assessment will include quantitative and qualitative information about the nature and extent of emotional problems, using various standardised assessments. We will consider some options here before going on to look at the use of self-monitoring systems.

Using Storyboards to Explore Social Cognition and Emotional Understanding

The Social Information Processing model, developed by Dodge and Frame (1982), offers a framework to understand how key social cognitive skills affect how we come to understand social experiences. The model also takes account of why individuals might interpret social events as they do, with consideration of a range of social cognitive skills such as perspective taking and empathy; the ability to judge others actions and intentions; the ability to choose a response; the ability to discriminate between helpful and unhelpful actions; and the impact of these actions. This process can offer an explanation of how both cognitive biases and cognitive deficits may translate to a particular behavioural response.

The Social Information Processing model influenced our research with people with intellectual disabilities and problems of aggression (Pert et al. 1999; Jahoda et al. 2006; Pert and Jahoda 2008). We used storyboards to explore views of imagined provocation and interpersonal conflict. We have found that storyboards are a flexible and useful tool that can be used in a clinical context to explore clients' emotional understanding and social cognitive skills; this can offer useful information when working with clients who may struggle to make sense of interpersonal experiences. The storyboards we have developed are short accessible stories represented by photographs, usually describing social interactions. Similar materials could quite easily be drawn up by a resourceful therapist to target the topics that are most relevant for their client. The story structure generally has three stages, with each stage represented by a photograph. The client is asked to comment on the characters' intentions, emotions, behaviour and actions (e.g. *why did she do that; how did it make her feel; why does she feel that way; what should she do?*) Alternatively, the format of the story can be self-referent, meaning that the client is asked to imagine themselves in the story (e.g. *how did it make you feel; why did you feel that way; what would you do?*).

As stated, the process can help identify particular cognitive characteristics or areas of cognitive difficulty, which in turn allows the therapist to adapt CBT accordingly or identify when CBT is perhaps not the best option. An added advantage is that storyboards can be a good way of engaging clients who are uncomfortable talking about their own experiences. Stories can act as an icebreaker and a helpful springboard to go on to discuss real-life experiences.

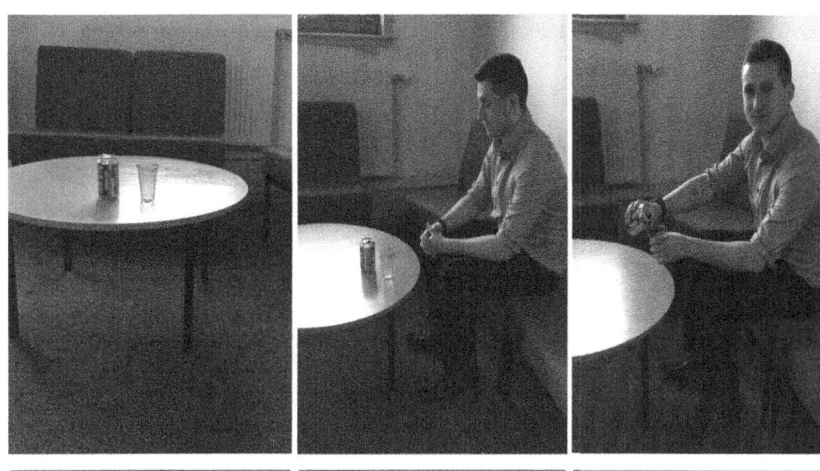

| Peter leaves his drink on the table in the café and goes to the toilet. | When he comes back someone is sitting with his drink | Peter says 'that's mine', but the guy ignores him and pours the drink into his glass. |

The following short extract is taken from an interview with John, using the storyboard called 'Stealing Your Drink', to explore his social understanding. John's response to questions highlights a discrepancy between his attribution of the character's intent ('*it was a mistake*'), and his chosen action ('*phone the Police*'), suggesting a possible difficulty with social reasoning or social problem solving.

Example Questions from Storyboard Stealing Your Drink

Therapist: Do you think he deliberately took the drink or was it a mistake?
Client: It was a mistake.
Therapist: How would you feel if that happened to you?
Client: I'd be angry.
Therapist: Why would you be angry?
Client: He's got my drink.
Therapist: What would you do when he takes your drink?
Client: I'd phone the Police.

The storyboard approach can also be used to demonstrate the link between thinking, feelings and action, in much the same way as the role play exercises we will discuss in the following chapters. There is scope to identify biases in thinking from themes that are shown in the interpretation of these stories, for example, a tendency to view others as having unfriendly intentions.

Standardised Assessments

The concept of measurement is central to the CBT approach. Usually this involves measuring the extent of the problem before, during and after therapy, using validated and reliable measures. Certainly when working in an National Health Service (NHS) context there is a drive towards consistent use of outcome measures within and across services to allow better quality control and contribute to audit and evaluation. In this context it is crucial that the measures are valid and reliable. Therapy outcome measures can be completed by the client or a third party, such as a family member or carer; however, there are clear advantages to using self-report assessments in CBT therapy. As things stand, there are relatively few standardised self-report measures that have been developed specifically for use with people who have intellectual disabilities (McGurk and Skelly 2006). The Glasgow Depression Scale (Cuthill et al. 2003) and the Glasgow Anxiety Scale (Mindham and Espie 2003) are two exceptions. Both have been validated for use with people with intellectual disabilities and have good reliability and validity. These are relatively short self-report measures (20 and 27 items) that explore specific targeted emotions experienced in the previous week, with each item rated on a three-point scale (never/sometimes/always). Usually the therapist will read the questions to the client with intellectual disabilities in a structured interview format. By reading aloud to the client, the questions can be incorporated more naturally into the clinical conversation to maintain the flow of sessions. Another self-report assessment specifically developed for the client group is the Anger Inventory (Rose and Gerson 2009).

One disadvantage of assessments that target one emotion is that these fail to take account of co-morbidity issues; yet, there is no agreed or widely used concept of generic outcomes (e.g. Skelly et al. 2006). The CORE-LD (Clinical Outcomes in Routine Evaluation-Learning Disabilities) is one of the few measures developed especially for the intellectual disability client group that measures broader generic outcomes as opposed to targeted emotions (Barton et al. 2008). Again this is a brief measure (14 items) and each item is illustrated by pictures to support understanding, with a three-point rating scale (not at all/sometimes/a lot).

Other standardised measures have been adapted from non-learning-disability sources, such as the Brief Symptom Inventory (Kellett et al. 2003, 2004), Inventory of Interpersonal Problems—32 (Kellett et al. 2005), Novaco Anger Scale (Novaco and Taylor 2004), Provocation Inventory (Novaco and Taylor 2004). Another assessment that is used relatively often is the Rosenberg Self-Esteem Scale (Davis et al. 2009), although this has not been adapted for use with people with intellectual disabilities.

Self-Monitoring and Diaries

In keeping with the assessment of outcomes, self-monitoring and recording is a fundamental component of CBT that can also help therapists and clients to keep track of progress. An added benefit for clients with intellectual disabilities is that diaries can help overcome memory problems. Generally CBT therapists introduce diaries during the first or second session, asking clients to keep a record of antecedents, emotions, thoughts and actions. Clearly, the process and format of diaries will require considerable adjustment when working with clients with intellectual disabilities.

Whatever approach is used it is important for the therapist to take time to talk the process through with the client and to practise completing the sheets. By ensuring that your client understands what is expected of them, it follows that they are more likely to complete the diaries between sessions. Taking time to talk through the approach also helps to identify whether the format used is suitable for your client and whether the therapist needs to take a different tack.

When clients lack the ability or confidence to complete the recordings on their own it might be suggested that they could complete them with the assistance of someone else. Once again, don't assume that a family member or worker will necessarily grasp what they are being asked to do or what the purpose is. For example, on a number of occasions when we have given clients recording sheets to complete with the help of a support worker, concerning their mood and activity, the diaries have been used to record incidents of challenging behaviour, (i.e. a list of what the support person feels the clients has done wrong during the week and what the worker wants the therapist to fix). Usually though, the main difficulty is to get clients to make recordings on a regular basis. Given that self-monitoring has generally been shown to be a helpful therapeutic tool in its own right (Moss-Morris et al. 2010), it is worth persisting.

Common Stumbling Blocks

Self-monitoring can seem like a pointless exercise when the therapist finds themselves reviewing diaries which haven't been filled out, lack the necessary information or fail to answer the questions asked. For therapists working with clients with intellectual disabilities there are a number of common stumbling blocks which often impact on the quality of information recorded. These broadly fall into two main categories of (i) problems relating to the clients' understanding and skills and (ii) problems linked with the ability to organise and self-manage the process. The underlying issues can include poor literacy and numeracy skills, poor emotional understanding, cognitive characteristics, memory problems, poor organisational skills and low motivation. We have already highlighted in Chap. 2 that planning and implementing routines can be a challenge for many clients with intellectual disabilities, particularly those with poor executive functioning.

Helpful Building Blocks: What You Can Do

In most cases self-monitoring is introduced at the outset of therapy. Yet at this early stage the therapist may not have a clear grasp of the client's capabilities. With this in mind, we suggest that the 'less is more' rule be followed, keeping diaries simple to avoid clients feeling overwhelmed or demoralised. It should be remembered that even clients with relatively good understanding may lack confidence with written tasks. By starting small you can pace the task according to the person's confidence and understanding, and improve compliance in the long run. More sophisticated methods can then be introduced in a better informed fashion, with less risk of misjudgement.

Problems Due to Cognitive Characteristics

In order to reduce the cognitive and literacy demands when completing diaries, a good place to start is by simplifying language and ensuring that all information is clear and unambiguous. It is worth checking your client's understanding of the vocabulary used, particularly the words used to describe emotions. Use your client's own terminology whenever possible (anxious/stressed/uptight/high). One of our clients referred to his depression as 'a dark cloud that rains on me' and discussing his 'cloud' was more meaningful to him than using unfamiliar terms such as 'depression' or 'depressed mood'.

In terms of presentation and layout, the therapist should avoid putting too much information on one page, as this can be overwhelming and increase confusion for clients with poor reading skills and poor eyesight. It is good practice to use large text and an easy read font. The layout should ensure that the key points stand out. Use visuals to aid understanding, such as the use of contrasting colours, pictures or symbols. These have the added advantage of being visually eye-catching and attention-grabbing. You can personalise diaries to suit the client, which also offers the opportunity to represent cultural and other diversity characteristics. Rating scales should also be carefully chosen according to ability, and a number of options will be considered later in this chapter.

Again, the principles of scaffolding learning are helpful. Therapists should use an experiential learning approach, working through diaries alongside the client to demonstrate how each question might be answered. By dedicating enough time to practise with the client, the therapist can get useful insights into underlying issues. By following this process we became aware of one client's embarrassment about her spelling and handwriting, and could reassure her that these are common concerns and unimportant. This also highlighted more general concerns the client had about how she is viewed by others.

When a client lacks literacy skills, teaching them to use a dictaphone and to audio record their mood and thoughts is an alternative option. Most mobile phones have cameras and clients and supporters could be asked to take photographs of themselves completing tasks they have planned to do. Many individuals with intellectual disabilities use features on their mobile phone even when they lack good literacy skills. It would even be possible to have a set of pre-recorded questions that clients answer.

Increasing Compliance

The therapist should establish when diaries should be filled out, perhaps anchoring this to a daily routine such as mealtimes or bedtime or a favourite television programme. The support of carers will often be crucial to get this routine up and running and to increase compliance. It might also overcome the common problem of a backlog of diaries being filled out hurriedly before each appointment, impacting on the quality of information given.

To enhance compliance, we have already highlighted the importance of agreeing on a clear rationale. It may seem obvious that clients should be informed of why they are keeping a diary, yet we have found that this can often be unclear. To demonstrate the importance of diaries the therapist should set aside adequate time to review their content during sessions. Interestingly, in a study checking the therapy fidelity of therapists using CBT with clients with ID, diaries were reviewed in only half of the sessions that were rated (Haddock et al. 2001).

Other small changes can have a big impact on compliance and organisation. To avoid clients losing sheets, or forgetting to bring diary sheets to sessions, it is often a good idea to use a booklet format or personalised folder rather than single paper sheets. This can make a surprising difference, perhaps as it gives the task more visibility and prestige. Also, using a folder allows the therapist to collate diary sheets chronologically to help clients keep track. A phone call can also be useful reminder for some people.

A summary of tips to improve the quality of self-monitoring are shown below.

Problems due to understanding and literacy	Problems with compliance, organisation and planning

Do this √
   Start small and build up gradually to ensure understanding
   Make sure written information is simple, clear and adapted to meet the needs of your client
   Make sure the structure and layout is clear
   Use colours (e.g. red for angry, blue for calm), pictures and symbols to aid understanding
   Use rating scales that suit ability and aid understanding with colour coding and visual aids
   Use mobile phones and voice recorders when appropriate
	Do this √
	   Take time to explain the purpose and benefits of the diaries at the outset
	   Suggest a daily routine for diaries and decide who will help
	   Use a folder or booklet rather than single sheets of paper
	   Personalise the diary to give a sense of ownership
	   Schedule a 'between session' reminder, such as a text message or a phone call

Choosing the Best Fit for Your Client

The best diary format will partly depend on the purpose of self-monitoring. In some cases, this might be to find out which emotions are being experienced by the client day to day (*How did I feel today?*). In other cases the purpose may be to identify the frequency of an identified emotion such as anxiety or anger. Or you may wish to establish the severity of a particular emotion, or identify the trigger events and coping response that followed. As noted earlier, the broad purpose of diaries should be made clear to clients and carers, as this will enhance compliance.

The content and format of questions asked will vary in complexity depending on the ability of the client and the purpose of the monitoring. Open-ended questions (*How are you feeling?*) should only be used with clients who have sufficient literacy skills to write an open-ended response. A multiple choice format, where clients choose from a set of options, might be more helpful, such as a daily tick box diary (*tick √ the box to show*

how you feel: angry ☐; *uptight* ☐; *happy* ☐). Providing options to choose from in this way overrides the need for a written response. Clients' understanding can be further supported by pictures of facial expression of emotion to accompany each item.

For some clients self monitoring may be limited to a simple frequency check that is completed each time they experience an identified emotion (*put a sticker in the box every time you feel sad*), whereas others may be able to rate the severity of their emotion (*a little bit sad/quite sad/really sad*). The addition of contextual information (*where were you; what were you doing*) can also be added if the client has adequate literacy skills.

If you are unsure of your client's capabilities, often it is best to start with a relatively straightforward option such as recording the frequency of emotions each day. This establishes a baseline for the extent of the client's problem and also introduces the client to the idea of 'tuning in' and monitoring their internal states. The therapist can then use this information during sessions to 'drill down' to establish the associated unhelpful thoughts and trigger events, perhaps using role play and other methods.

As already discussed above, the therapist should make use of technologies when developing self monitoring systems. Most people with literacy skills have mobile phones, and these are usually brought to sessions.

Choosing Rating Scales: How Much and How Often

When asking clients to rate 'how much' of a problem they have, or 'how often' an emotion occurs, again it is important to adapt the format to suit your client's level of understanding.

1. Visual analogue scales are a flexible method that can be used to grade the severity (*a little bit, quite a bit, a lot*) or the frequency (*never, sometimes, always*) of an emotion. These simple ratings can offer a helpful way of tracking change. The use of visual analogue scales can be supported with pictures indicating the meaning of the scale. The scale can

be either unipolar (*a bit stressed,* <-----> *very stressed*) or bipolar (calm <-----> anxious). There is some evidence that children and adults tend to apply bipolar constructs to their experience (*strong/weak; happy/sad*); however, unipolar constructs are arguably more straightforward. Unipolar scales can start with the absence of a dimension and move to the maximum level (*not angry* <------> *very angry*). Colour can be used to emphasise the changing dimension. As usual, any rating measures should be practised within sessions to make sure these are understood.

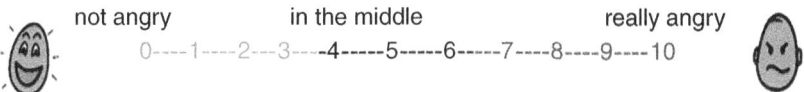

not angry   in the middle   really angry
0----1----2---3---**4-----5-----6-----7**----8----9----10

2. The bar chart is a very commonly used rating system, which appears to be favoured by researchers working in the intellectual disabilities field. It has been used in standardised assessments developed for people with intellectual disabilities (Glasgow Anxiety Scale and Glasgow Depression Scale and Core-learning disability (LD)). Most often clients are asked to choose from three graded options (*never/sometimes/always*) on an increasing scale, although some clients will cope with four or five options. Similar to visual analogue scales, unipolar (*a little bit sad/quite sad/very sad*) or bipolar constructs (*calm/in the middle/stressed*) can be used. Pictures and colour coding will support understanding.

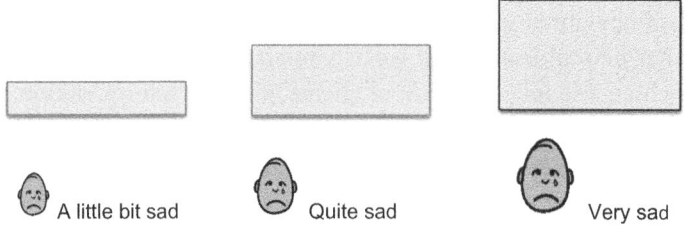

A little bit sad   Quite sad   Very sad

3. Tick box frequency charts don't require the ability to use graded systems, as clients are asked to simply tick a box, or put a sticker in the box, each time the problem occurs.

4. Forced choice is another option wherein you can also ask clients to choose an emotion from a range of options provided as shown below.

Tick a box ✓ to say how you feel.

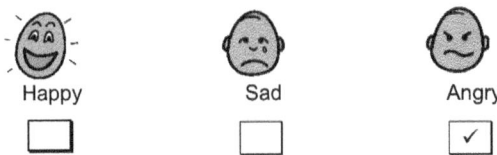

Self-Perceptions

Self-identity and views of self are core issues in CBT. Given that many clients will have experience of being in a subordinate role in many, if not most, relationships, we find it helpful to look broadly at clients' views of self and 'self in relation to others', drawing from work carried out by Peter Trower, who developed this model in research carried out with people with a diagnosis of psychosis. Trower and Chadwick (1995) drew from social cognitive theory to devise a three-part model which incorporates (i) views of self, (ii) views of others and (iii) views of 'how others see me'. We used this framework for clients with ID, showing that additional insights can be achieved to support formulation. We will hear more about this model in Chap. 5. It is also important to keep in mind how common life experiences such as stigmatisation and lack of autonomy might impact on clients' views of self, as highlighted in Chaps. 1 and 2 of this book.

Another helpful framework is Kelly's personal construct theory (Kelly 1955), which also takes account of clients' views of self in relation to others. Comparing one's 'self' with an 'ideal self' can offer helpful insights when setting therapeutic goals. A repertory grid approach is used to explore how clients make sense of experiences. Dougal Hare and colleagues discuss the advantages of using repertory grids with clients who have intellectual disabilities, particularly as the process is person centred and doesn't aim to compare clients against a 'perceived norm'. Hare et al. (2011) describe how this model was used in the case of one client, Ann, who had anger problems and an intellectual disability. The assessment process showed that Ann's view of herself was quite different from the views of her support team who saw her as 'mentally ill' and of limited ability. In contrast, Ann viewed herself as being more able than her peers and sought to align herself with individuals who don't have an intellectual disability. In short, the repertory grid highlighted Ann's discomfort with being labelled and patronised, which contributed to Ann's anger, and led to further conflict.

A useful screening tool when exploring clients' self-image is the Butler Self Image Profile (Butler and Gasson 2004). It uses a relatively 'easy read' format and is short and quick to administer. The items are well balanced to include positive and negative qualities. The checklist can be used to introduce discussion about the client's self-identity and has a helpful focus on 'How I am' compared with 'How I want to be' in line with the personal construct approach. This can offer a very fruitful line of enquiry at the early stages of therapy.

We have tried to highlight how the route that therapy takes in early CBT sessions will vary greatly depending on an assortment of factors, including the client's motivation, communication ability, social and emotional understanding and their engagement with the therapy process. Once the therapist has successfully established rapport and listened to the client's own personal account of their problem, she will also have gauged the most suitable pace and depth of clinical discussions and selected appropriate standardised assessments and monitoring systems to suit the needs of the client. This offers a good foundation for the next stage of assessment; socialising your client to the CBT model and working towards formulation, which are covered in the next two chapters.

To demonstrate the journey taken from assessment through to formulation and intervention, we will follow the case of Jean, introduced below, over the course of the next two chapters.

> **Jean: Background Information and Initial Assessment**
>
> *Referral: Jean was referred by her community nurse for help with significant anxiety problems and low mood. Jean has been seen by a psychiatrist for the past five years and has been prescribed medication to be*

taken as required when she plans to leave the house.

Background and current circumstances: After attending her local primary school for a year, Jean was transferred to a special school for people with intellectual disabilities. She moved on to another special school when she reached secondary school stage. She enjoyed school and reported having friends there and taking advantage of the extracurricular activities on offer, including several trips abroad. However, she was bussed across the city from her home to school and had little contact with her school friends outside school. She remained socially isolated at home and knew few of the other children in her neighbourhood. In fact, she reported being called names by local children when she was playing outside with her younger brother, who was very protective of her.

When Jean left school she attended a college course for people with intellectual disabilities for two years. Since then she has had very limited daily activity, apart from a literacy class once a week and a drama group. Her one regular evening activity is a swimming group for people with intellectual disabilities. On some occasions, her cousin has taken her to live music concerts and to the cinema. However, she has become increasingly reluctant to go out to concerts, after she panicked when her cousin took her to seats high up in the auditorium. Jean had to leave during the performance which made her feel 'upset and stupid'. She also used to go to the cinema with a friend from her drama group but this stopped around the time she panicked at the concert.

Jean lives at home with her parents. Her brother and his family live nearby and have regular contact with Jean. Her father is a bus driver and her mother does not work and regards her main role as looking after Jean. They are a close family and Jean's parents involve her in their social activities, which mainly revolve round a large extended family.

Presenting problem: Jean has become highly anxious when she leaves the family home, particularly if it involves travel to new locations or where there is a view of open spaces and hills. She can also become anxious in busy locations like shops and restaurants. In the past, Jean used to accompany her parents on family holidays and outings, including abroad. However, this stopped after Jean had become very distressed on a flight to visit her aunt and uncle in America and she remained in a highly anxious state during their stay, in anticipation of the flight home.

Assessment and clinical interview: The Glasgow Depression and Anxiety scales were completed with Jean and time was spent talking with her about her difficulties. Over the first three sessions she also kept self-report sheets about her level of anxiety. Jean has very limited literacy skills and was therefore unable to write about her experiences in detail but the recordings she kept helped to identify situations that she had found anxiety provoking and the coping mechanisms that she used. At Jean's request, her mother sat in for the whole of the first session and joined us for the final 15 minutes of the following two sessions.

Jean's scores on the Glasgow Anxiety and Depression scales were highly clinically significant. Looking qualitatively at the pattern of her responses on the assessments, it emerged that she worried a great deal about her family and what would happen to her in the future, as well as what other people thought about her. Jean also had a range of specific fears or phobias and disliked busy places, heights and wide open spaces. Jean said she experienced strong physiological symptoms of anxiety, in particular she felt 'shaky, breathless and had a racing heart' in anxiety-provoking situations. Her low mood seemed to stem from a general sense of distress and hopelessness about her current situation.

Jean's mother was worried that Jean would find therapy distressing and that the therapist would fail to realise the nature of her difficulties and set unrealistic goals for her.

We will pick up Jean's case in the following chapter.

> **Key Points**
>
> 1. As clients rarely refer themselves for therapy, their expectation, motivation and possible misconceptions should be addressed at the outset.
> 2. The usual process of gathering relevant background information will take longer than usual, so the therapist should not set unrealistic expectations of what can be achieved in the first few assessment sessions.
> 3. Adjustments can be made to the pace of sessions, depth of questioning and the nature of the information conveyed according to clients' varying needs. The therapist has to adjust her own communication and interaction style rather than trying to 'improve' the client.
> 4. The route that therapy takes in early CBT sessions will vary greatly depending on an assortment of factors, including the client's motivation, communication ability, social and emotional understanding and cognitive style.
> 5. Self-report standardised assessments should be chosen to match the client's difficulties, and also their level of emotional understanding.
> 6. Creative methods can be used to adapt self-monitoring diaries and increase compliance.

References

Bachelor, A., & Horvarth, A. (1999). The therapeutic relationship. In M. A. Hubble, B. L. Duncan, & S. D. Miller (Eds.), *The heart and soul of change: What works in therapy* (pp. 133–178). Washington, DC: American Psychological Association.

Barton, P., Brooks, M., Davies, S., Flynn, T., & Wood, V. (2008). From CORE-OM to CORE-LD through participatory research. *Clinical Psychology and People with Learning Disabilities, 6*, 27–28. doi:10.1111/j.1468-3156.2007.00476.x.

Beutler, L. E., Machado, P. P., & Neufeldt, S. A. (1994). Therapist variables. In A. E. Bergin & S. L. Garfield (Eds.), *Handbook of psychotherapy and behaviour change* (4th ed., pp. 229–269). New York: Wiley.

Butler, R. J., & Gasson, S. L. (2004). *Self image profile for adults (SIP-adult)*. London: Pearsons Clinical.

Cuthill, F. M., Espie, C. A., & Cooper, S.-A. (2003). Development and psychometric properties of the Glasgow depression scale for people with a learning disability: Individual and carer supplement versions. *British Journal of Psychiatry, 182*, 347–353.

Davis, C., Kellett, S., & Beail, N. (2009). Utility of the Rosenberg self-esteem scale. *American Journal of Intellectual Development Disability, 114*(3), 172–178.

Delsignore, A., & Schnyder, U. (2007). Control expectancies as predictors of psychotherapy outcome: A systematic review. *British Journal of Clinical Psychology, 46*(4), 467–483.

Dodge, K. A., & Frame, C. L. (1982). Social cognitive biases and deficits in aggressive boys. *Child Development, 53*, 620–635.

Dunn, A., Stenfert Kroese, B., Thomas, G., McGarry, A., & Drew, P. (2006). Are you allowed to say that? Using video materials to provide accessible information about psychology services. *British Journal of Learning Disabilities, 34*(4), 215–219.

Eckman, P. (1993). Facial expression and emotion. *American Psychologist, 48*(4), 384–392.

Gilbert, P., & Leahy, R. L. (2007). Introduction and overview: Basic issues in the therapeutic relationship. In P. Gilbert & R. L. Leahey (Eds.), *The therapeutic relationship in the cognitive behavioral psychotherapies*. London: Routledge.

Haddock, G., Devane, S., Bradshaw, T., McGovern, J., Tarrier, N., Kinderman, P., Baguley, I., Lancashire, S., & Harris, N. (2001). An investigation into the psychometric properties of the cognitive therapy scale for psychosis (CTS-Psy). *Behavioural and Cognitive Psychotherapy, 29*, 221–233.

Hare, D. J., Searson, R., & Knowles, R. (2011). Real listening – Using personal construct assessment with people with intellectual disabilities: Two case studies. *British Journal of Learning Disabilities, 39*(3), 190–197.

Jahoda, A., Pert, C., & Trower, P. (2006). Frequent aggression and attribution of hostile intent in people with mild to moderate intellectual disabilities: An empirical investigation. *American Journal on Mental Retardation, 111*, 90–99.

Joyce, A. S., & Piper, W. E. (1998). Expectancy, the therapeutic alliance, and treatment outcome in short term individual psychotherapy. *Psychotherapy Research, 5*, 49–62.

Kellett, S. C., Beail, N., Newman, D. W., & Frankish, P. (2003). Utility of the Brief Symptom Inventory (BSI) in the assessment of psychological distress. *Journal of Applied Research in Intellectual Disabilities, 16*, 127–135.

Kellett, S. C., Beail, N., Newman, D. W., & Hawes, A. (2004). The factor structure of the Brief Symptom Inventory: Intellectual disability evidence. *Clinical Psychology and Psychotherapy, 11*, 275–281.

Kellett, S., Beaill, N., & Newman, D. W. (2005). Measuring interpersonal problems in people with mental retardation. *American Journal on Mental Retardation, 110*(2), 136–144.

Kelly, G. A. (1955). *The psychology of personal constructs*. New York: Norton.

Kilbane, A., & Jahoda, A. (2011). Therapy expectations: Preliminary exploration and measurement in adults with intellectual disabilities. *Journal of Applied Research in Intellectual Disability, 24*, 528–542.

Lindsay, W. R., Tinsley, S., Beail, N., Hastings, R. P., Jahoda, A., Taylor, J. L., & Hatton, C. (2015). A preliminary controlled trial of a trans-diagnostic programme for cognitive behaviour therapy with adults with intellectual disability. *Journal of Intellectual Disability Research, 59*(4), 360–369.

McDonald, J., Sinason, V., & Hollins, S. (2003). An interview study of people with learning disabilities experience of, and satisfaction with, group analytic therapy. *Psychology and Psychotherapy Theory Research and Practice, 76*, 433–453.

McGurk, K. A., & Skelly, A. (2006). A quick guide for psychologists working in learning disability on the available clinical outcome measures currently in use. *The Bulletin of the Faculty for People with Intellectual Disabilities, 12*(1), 28–45.

Mindham, J., & Espie, C. A. (2003). Glasgow anxiety scale for people with an intellectual disability (GAS-ID): Development and psychometric properties of a new measure for use with people with mild intellectual disability. *Journal of Intellectual Disability Research, 47*(1), 22–30.

Moss-Morris, R., McAlpine, L., Didsbury, L. P., & Spence, M. J. (2010). A randomized controlled trial of a cognitive behavioural therapy-based self-management intervention for irritable bowel syndrome in primary care. *Psychological Medicine, 40*(1), 85–94.

Novaco, R. W., & Taylor, J. L. (2004). Assessment of anger and aggression in male offenders with developmental disabilities. *Psychological Assessment, 16*, 42–50.

Pert, C., & Jahoda, A. (2008). Social goals and conflict strategies of individuals with mild to moderate intellectual disabilities who present problems of aggression. *Journal of Intellectual Disability Research, 52*, 393–403.

Pert, C., Jahoda, A., & Squire, J. (1999). Attribution of intent and role-taking: Cognitive factors as mediators of aggression with people who have mental retardation. *American Journal on Mental Retardation, 104*(5), 399–409.

Pert, C., Jahoda, A., Stenfert Kroese, B., Trower, P., Dagnan, D., & Selkirk, M. (2013). Cognitive behavioural therapy from the perspective of clients with mild intellectual disabilities: A qualitative investigation of process issues. *Journal of Intellectual Disability Research, 57*, 359–369.

Reed, J., & Clements, J. (1989). Assessing the understanding of emotional states in a population of adolescents and young adults with mental handicaps. *Journal of Mental Deficiency, Research, 33*, 229–233.

Rose, J. L., & Gerson, D. F. (2009). Assessing anger in people with intellectual disability. *Journal of Intellectual Developmental Disability, 34*(2), 116–122.

Skelly, A., Delicata, J., & D'Antonio, M.-L. (2006). Are CTPLDs effective? Use of the HoNOS-LD and LEC as outcome measures in community teams. *Clinical Psychology and People with Learning Disabilities, 7*, 28–33.

Trower, P., & Chadwick, P. (1995). Pathways to defense of the self: A theory of two types of paranoia. *Clinical Psychology Science and Practice, 2*(3), 263–278.

5

The First Stage of Therapy

This chapter picks up on the client's journey through therapy after the first few sessions have been completed. By this stage rapport with the therapist should be established and clients should have a clear idea why they are meeting with the therapist and a grasp of what happens in therapy sessions. One of the differences of working with individuals who have intellectual disabilities is that it often takes longer for the therapist to acquire the necessary information to produce a formulation than it would when working in a typical adult mental health outpatient setting. Another difference is that it can prove challenging to socialise clients to have an understanding of the CBT model early in therapy. Therefore, taking a pragmatic approach, where the end of the first stage of therapy is marked by the delivery of a formulation, we consider that this will usually take four to five sessions. So this chapter takes us up to the delivery of the formulation, when the therapist and client develop an agreed formulation or a first plan for working together. However, it is worth bearing in mind that when working with clients there is likely to be some overlap between the different stages of therapy. On occasion, it might be important to begin therapeutic work at an early stage when there are issues that it would be sensible to address in a more timely way.

Before Moving Forward: Taking Stock About the Model to Be Used

Therapists using CBT are aiming to reduce clients' emotional distress by helping them to change their maladaptive ways of thinking and behaving in the world. In Rational Emotive Behavioural Therapy (REBT) an important distinction is made between inferences and evaluations (Trower et al. 2015). Whilst people's inferences or perceptions of events may or may not be accurate, depending on their personal biases, it is the evaluations that they attach to them that cause distress. The evaluations are value judgements about the inferences people make. One way of explaining this distinction would be in terms of the judgements that people might make when observing an event happening to others as compared to being personally affected. Events observed from a distance can be interpreted in a dispassionate fashion or may not be emotionally affecting. When we are personally involved as an actor then we evaluate what the event means for *ourselves* at an *emotional level*. For example, lack of success at a job interview might result in me inferring that I had done badly. My distress is caused by my evaluation that I am a failure.

The distinction between inferences and evaluations is important when working with people who are facing emotional difficulties that are based in reality. Someone with an intellectual disability may be right to believe that other people are staring at them or that they need help with everyday tasks. What may be important to challenge are hurtful self-evaluations arising from these experiences, such as seeing themselves as worthless or stupid.

Adapting CBT to the Needs of an ID Client

Of course it goes without saying that each therapist will bring their own unique style and ways of relating into the therapy room. The therapist's value base and life experiences will also affect interactions with clients. Padesky points out that the progress made in CBT will be enhanced or limited by the beliefs of the therapist. Indeed, one might assume that this is true irrespective of the therapeutic approach.

Considering how therapist variables might interact with client charactersitics, highlights the need for a framework to help navigate these therapeutic dynamics. An example might be the therapist who places a high value on professional boundaries and gets thrown off course when a socially disinhibited client asks him or her a personal question. Or perhaps a therapist who relies on a well-planned and structured approach to his or her sessions finds it difficult to adjust when the client repeatedly changes the topic. Whilst neither therapist's style is incorrect, the interaction of therapist and client factors is clearly a problem.

After spending the first few sessions obtaining information and getting to know and interacting with the client, it is a good time for the therapist to reflect on modifications that might need to be made for therapeutic work. The skill of the CBT therapist in services for people with intellectual disabilities is to modify the CBT model to overcome, as far as possible, any obstacles to therapy progress. A helpful framework for adapting CBT for use with a range of diverse client groups that works for people with intellectual disabilities is offered by Westbrook et al. (2010). They chart the possible interactions of client characteristics, therapist characteristics, client context, therapist/service context and how this fits with the CBT model. Crucially, the focus is on the *interface* between these variables and how they can be accommodated in a CBT model. This offers a more helpful standpoint than focusing simply on client 'deficits'. Taking account of how these factors work together helps the therapist pinpoint which aspects of therapy may need to be modified on a case-by-case basis. To show how this framework might apply to our clients we have populated each of the five subdomains with some common issues that arise when working with clients with intellectual disabilities.

Common Client Characteristics

- Cognitive skills such as attention and memory ability.
- Self-regulation skills and perspective-taking ability.

- Clients' ability to self-monitor, self-report and distinguish thoughts and emotions.
- Communication ability and conversational skills, turn taking and listening skills.
- Self-efficacy and acquiescence.

Client Context

- The client's experiences of being excluded, bullied or stigmatised. Other negative social experiences such as being patronised or overlooked.
- Extensive input from a range of health and social care providers, which may colour expectations of therapy and lead to low self-efficacy.
- Lifelong support from a loving family but limited opportunity for a sense of adulthood.
- Few social contacts (e.g. it is less common for clients to be married, have children or sexual relationships). Lack of meaningful occupation and structure in life.

Therapist Characteristics

- The therapist's familiarity with the client group.
- Values, beliefs and attitudes of the therapist, and their assumptions about disability.
- The therapist's use of reflective practice.
- Flexibility of the therapeutic approach.
- The ability to adapt communication to meet the client's needs, including using visual aids, talking mats which use pictures to help people express their views and so on.

Service Requirements

- Location of appointments and the flexibility allowed to overcome difficulties clients may experience in getting to appointments.

- The scope to work long term with clients who require more time to settle into therapy.
- Good links with social care service providers, social work departments and commissioning teams.
- Scope for multidisciplinary working.

The following case example shows how the process can help explore adjustments to CBT with a client who has a mild intellectual disability.

The framework reminds us of the need to look beyond client characteristics when seeking to resolve difficulties that arise in therapy.

> **A Case Example**
>
> Marie is aged 27 years and has a mild intellectual disability. She has been referred for anxiety problems.
>
> *Client Characteristics.* Marie's speech is impaired by articulation problems which worsens when she in anxious. Despite Marie's problems with expressive communication, her understanding of what is said appears to be good. When given the time to do so, Marie can reflect on her experiences and describe her emotions. However, she has a tendency to acquiesce and seek approval from others.
>
> *Client Context.* Marie lives in shared accommodation with two other service users. Her support hours have recently been reduced, meaning that opportunities for 1:1 time are now limited. A member of Marie's staff team has accompanied her to therapy sessions. Marie has had limited autonomy in her life and has lived in shared supported accommodation throughout her adult life.
>
> *Therapist Characteristics.* The therapist has limited experience of working with clients who have an intellectual disability. She has gathered most of the assessment information from Marie's support worker as she has struggled to understand Marie's speech. The therapist would appear to have focused too much on gathering background information, essentially asking Marie's carer for a series of 'facts' about the client. This focus on the carer may have resulted in Marie being even more passive in sessions, making it difficult to build meaningful engagement and rapport.
>
> *Therapist/Service Context.* The therapist works in a multidisciplinary team that uses standardised assessment protocols. The team is based in a health centre and mainly offers clinic appointments at the centre. Marie does not have support staff on shift to accompany her to sessions at the set clinic time. It is agreed that the therapist should phone Marie's service provider to discuss alternative arrangements.
>
> *CBT Model.* Marie's lack of participation means that there is little scope for the therapist to explore thoughts and feelings.

> **Revised Action Plan**
>
> The therapist decides to focus more on relationship building in the next few sessions and involve Marie more fully by using DVD and visual materials to support her communication. It is hoped that this process will also offer the opportunity to establish a more collaborative relationship and assessment of whether CBT is the most appropriate way of helping Marie.
>   To overcome the problem Marie has with attending clinic appointments, the therapist decides to arrange home visits for future sessions. The standard protocol for assessment is reviewed to improve accessibility for clients with intellectual disabilities.

Socialising into the Model

The A-B-C model provides a relatively straightforward way of explaining CBT. One idea is that potential clients need to understand the links between events (A), thoughts about the events (B) and resulting emotions and behaviour (C), before they can begin therapy proper. To this end, assessments of clients' abilities to make A-B-C links have been developed for people with intellectual disabilities, as well as training packages to help them acquire the capacity to make these discriminations. As described in Chap. 3, efforts to assess and train these skills might prove to be an effective preparatory phase of therapy (Bruce et al. 2010). For the moment though, we would like to propose a rather different starting point: working with clients' own accounts of emotive events. This is a similar idea to working with 'hot cognitions'. In other words, when we talk about events which still have a strong emotional trace, we are more likely to give an account of what happened that includes an interpretation of events, how it made us feel and think about ourselves, and what we ended up doing and were left feeling. Thus, rather than regarding the ability to make A-B-C links as a new skill to be learned, the aim is to help clients reflect on their own interpretation of events they describe and their emotional and behavioural reactions. The aim of CBT is to tap into naturally occurring cognitive processes and to make them explicit or to bring them to consciousness. Working with clients' direct experience makes the process less abstract and more meaningful and relevant for the client; it's about trying to build on something that they can do rather than making it something new they need to learn. Ultimately, the aim is the same, to help clients recognise and tune into the impact of certain thoughts on their emotional lives but the process is different.

Hebblethwaite et al. (2011) compared people with and without intellectual disabilities' ability to talk about their thoughts and feelings in relation to real-life events and their ability to complete a formal assessment of A-B-C links (Dagnan and Chadwick 1997). Dagnan and Chadwick's formal assessment asks people to complete A-B-C links about a series of hypothetical situations. This formal measure can provide helpful insights into people's inferences and evaluations but the questions can be quite demanding. For example, one of the items is 'You are in bed one night and you hear a loud noise downstairs (A—event). You feel happy (C—resulting emotion). What would you be thinking or saying to yourself (mediating thought)?' The answer might be 'my flat mate has got back from his holiday'. In contrast, Hebblethwaite, Jahoda and Dagnan's semi-structured interview about real-life events involved asking the person to recall an incident which still has a strong emotional trace ('still bugs you') when they thought about it. The person was asked to hold that emotion in mind when they talked through what happened. The participants were then asked about their view of what happened (inferences) and the effect it had on them (evaluation).

The participants with intellectual disabilities were poorer than their non-disabled peers on both tasks. However, they fared better when the researchers used semi-structured interviews to talk about a real-life event that mattered to them. All of the participants with an intellectual disability were able to report their emotions and evaluative beliefs in relation to the incidents they recalled. However, a number of participants struggled to offer an explanation of why they thought an event had happened (inferences), whereas those without disabilities often offered several explanations. Let's take the example of a participant talking about a row they had had with someone. They might say that they felt really angry and they felt they were being treated 'like rubbish'. When asked what had happened, those with an intellectual disability might have struggled to go beyond saying that the other person was 'nasty', whereas those without an intellectual disability often gave several explanations. For instance, they might have said the other person was behaving badly to try and pass on the blame for their own mistakes or it was because they were a bad-tempered person or perhaps they behaved badly because they were under stress due to personal problems. If people with an intellectual disability find it hard to provide an explanation of events then it might be even harder to imagine taking a different view, associated with a different kind of evaluation or feeling. Thus, it may always not be easy to work with clients with an intellectual disability to help them take a different view of events.

How we made these A-B-C links explicit with Jean, the client we introduced at the end of Chap. 4, is shown below.

Making A-B-C Links with Jean

When reviewing how Jean had been getting on since we had last met, she said that she had become very 'uptight and panicky' when she had gone out for a meal with her parents. When I asked her to tell me what had happened, she described feeling 'uptight' when she went into the restaurant because it was busy (Jean had said in the first session that she became anxious on crowded buses). We used thought bubbles when talking about what happened when she was in the restaurant, drawn on a large piece of paper. She said that when the waiter came over to take their order she began to feel even more uptight and anxious. She said that she thought the waiter was staring at her and it made her feel 'terrible'. I then asked her about the reason the waiter was staring at her and she said that the waiter was thinking 'you shouldn't be here'. We then went on to talk about what she wanted to do when she felt so uptight. Jean said that she wanted to get out of the restaurant and go straight home, which would make her feel 'safe' and 'better'. When I asked what she did when she thought people were staring at her she said, 'don't look (at them)'.

We then used the pictures and thought bubbles that we had drawn to talk through the A-B-C links and how her underlying anxiety about going into the busy restaurant (Activating Event) led to the butterflies in her stomach and a racing heart (Consequences). In turn, her sense of panic about these physical symptoms of panic contributed to her thoughts that the waiter was staring at her and didn't want her to be there (didn't like her/was against her), which was 'terrible' (Beliefs). This made her feel even more uptight. She wanted to avoid eye contact and escape from the restaurant and get home, where she felt safe (Consequences).

We then took advantage of the thought bubbles we had produced to discuss how 'the thoughts in your head can affect what you feel'. We started by talking about other reasons that the waiter might have been looking towards her and whether or not he was really staring. Jean found it difficult to think of another reason why the waiter would have been looking at her and just kept saying that she thought the waiter was being 'nasty' and then just said 'I don't know', when she was pressed further. So we role-played being in the café and she took the part of the waitress, taking orders and looking after the customers. Afterwards, when she was asked 'what would be your job if someone was waiting to served', she said that the waiter is there to help customers. She agreed that this meant part of their job was to keep an eye on customers to make sure they are okay. We then used the thought bubbles to talk through what she would think and feel if she thought the waiter was just making sure she was 'okay'. She said that she would feel 'better'. She also realised that she did not know whether the waiter had been looking round at other people or not, because she was trying not to look at him. In turn, this led to a homework task where Jean was asked to look at the waiters the next time she went to a café or restaurant, to observe how they did their jobs and how often they looked round to check on customers.

Tapping into Clients' Thoughts and Underlying Schema or Views of Self

During the initial assessment phase, it may be possible to gain insight into the thoughts and self-perceptions of some clients with intellectual disabilities using tried and tested methods developed from general adult work. This includes downward chaining, where the therapist asks 'if then' type questions about the client's inferences, to tap into their underlying beliefs. For example, if a client tells the therapist that that they feel left out of family social events, you might ask them 'if that happens how are they treating you?' They might say 'like they don't want me' and then therapist would ask another 'what if' question. 'If you think they don't want you, how does that make you feel?' and the client might reply 'like I'm rubbish'.

Unfortunately, eliciting people's underlying cognitions and helping them to grasp the A-B-C links will be tricky with most clients. However, one important starting point is to be alert to what clients say and the kind of themes that emerge over the first phase of therapy. Even though clients may talk about different events, there may be common concerns. The therapist might be able to pick up that the client has a negative sense of self, a heightened perception of threat or beliefs about unfair treatment.

There are different ways of helping to elicit clients' thoughts and to make the A-B-C links more concrete. One frequently described approach is to use drawings and thought bubbles, as described with Jean above. An alternative approach is to role-play emotive situations with the client and stop them at crucial moments (you can use a TV remote control to indicate when to 'freeze' the role play by pretending to press the 'stop' button) to ask them what they are feeling, thinking and how they might behave. Again, you can use thought bubbles to draw out the thoughts and feeling people describe. The advantage of role play or acting is that it gives clients an active part to play in the session. You are not asking them to reflect on past events but to talk about a role play that's happening in the here and now. For instance, if someone has an anger problem and is quick to respond aggressively when they think they are being put down by a member of staff, the therapist can ask, what did it feel like when I said 'we need to get the kitchen cleaned up now'? 'How did you think I was treating you?' It is also possible to change roles and for the person to play the staff member, which in itself can be a useful way of helping the person to consider other possible reasons why the worker behaved in the way she did. Of course events are often dynamic and unfolding, and the use of techniques like role play (shifting perspective) can also help to illustrate how these processes work, such as conflicts leading to the breakdown in relationships and further conflict. Showing how different characters think and feel as events unfold might prove particularly helpful for individuals on the autistic spectrum, who have limited theory of mind.

Another reason for swapping roles is that some clients will find it too threatening or emotive to imagine themselves in difficult situations. If the client does not want to be part of a role play at all then it might be possible to invite a support person or another professional colleague to join the session and the client can be asked to direct the role play or tell the actors what to do. The therapist can stop at appropriate moments to ask the client 'what am I thinking now' and 'how does that make me feel?' As with the thought bubbles, it is possible to role-play a number of different versions of the same event, changing how the client is thinking or behaving.

It may also become apparent that an individual's distress is related to a realistic appraisal of events. As discussed in Chap. 2, care has to be taken to avoid assuming that the distress people report is necessarily due to distorted perceptions. Someone like Jean might well experience discriminatory treatment, including being stared at, with a negative impact on her sense of self.

Other concerns can remain unspoken. For example, sexuality is one subject that is often overlooked. In the otherwise excellent Glasgow Depression Scale (Cuthill et al. 2003), no mention is made of sexual interest, a factor included in all general adult depression scales. In my experience it is not uncommon for clients to have unspoken sexual concerns that emerge as therapy progresses. Being mindful of these issues means that the therapist can be careful to ensure that the client has an opportunity to talk about these oft-ignored topics.

The Way You Think

When seeking to grasp clients' evaluations it's not just their judgements about themselves or other people that matter, it's also their thinking styles. The kind of thinking that is thought to be maladaptive by CBT theorists is when it is rigidly negative or when there is a tendency to generalise from limited information. Even ordinary events, like when a support worker visits and suggests doing some tidying up, might feel devastating or catastrophic, for example, 'they must think I'm a bad person' or 'they're always picking on me and trying to put me down'. These types of errors not only lead clients to misinterpret events but they can misguide and restrict someone's actions.

Clients' thinking styles are likely to emerge when we begin to examine how events are perceived. Sometimes clients' thinking styles are not immediately obvious and will only emerge with careful questioning. In our research with people who have intellectual disabilities who are frequently aggressive, we asked participants to imagine themselves responding to conflict aggressively and submissively. We found that those with and without aggression held subtly different views (Kirk et al. 2008). Interestingly, both groups shared similar views about responding aggressively. Where the groups differed was that the aggressive participants found the idea of being submissive intolerable. In other words, the aggressive participants could not cope with the idea of being seen as weak by others. Establishing clients' thinking styles and the role this plays in their difficulties can be just as important as teasing out the content of cognitions.

Understanding Distress

Just like most of us, clients with intellectual disabilities are often distressed by their distress and can find it difficult to make sense of what is happening to them. Clients may say 'I just want to be myself again'. Another source of secondary distress for some clients is due to poor emotional regulation skills, leading them to feel that they are not in control of their feelings. Psycho-education can be immensely helpful at an early stage of therapy. For example, it can be reassuring for clients to know that their difficulties with concentration are linked to their depression. For those with anxiety problems, the flight or fight responses can be explained in simple terms. It might allow someone with agoraphobia to make sense of their overwhelming somatic symptoms and wish to escape to safety, when they panic in a crowded supermarket. Realising that panic is an understandable human reaction to perceived threat means that the client knows they are not alone in facing such difficulties. Offering these kinds of explanations may also help the client and therapist to build a common language and frame of reference to use when working on emotional problems. Care needs to be taken, however, as abstract explanations can leave clients with intellectual disabilities utterly confused. Explanations of the fight and fight response involving cave men fighting sabre-toothed tigers are rarely helpful, in our experience. Make sure that even apparently simple explanations are accessible and relevant to the individuals concerned.

Just as the therapist might want to help the client understand their emotional difficulties, they also need to avoid pathologising ordinary reactions to difficult life events like bereavement. Most therapists will have had a recently bereaved individual with intellectual disabilities referred for help because of their distress. In fact, I have even had individuals referred for help before they have been bereaved because it was anticipated that they would have difficulties coping. CBT therapy cannot replace close confiding relationships and timely and sensitive support from others (McRitchie et al. 2013). Perhaps in these instances it is the support workers who need to learn how to cope with clients' distress, to listen to them and stay alongside them when they cry.

The therapist should try to be non-judgemental in their approach when seeking to help clients understand their difficulties and be aware of their own biases. By this we mean that it would be mistaken to assume a certain set of beliefs or motivations on the part of the client. For example, don't assume that a client referred for anger management necessarily holds pro-social views and wishes to have better control over their anger. The client may not believe they have a difficulty or believe that their anger is helpful for them. Knowing what people actually think allows the therapist to find the right starting point for therapy.

The Role of Emotion

Taking clients' emotional experience seriously is a core aspect of CBT. Trower et al. (2015) draw on REBT to argue that negative emotions should not just be considered as symptoms of distress or mental health difficulties. They are part of being human so CBT therapy should not be about eliminating negative emotions as if they are a symptom of an illness. A starting point for therapy is often to help clients with intellectual disabilities to realise that their feelings are normal. If a client expresses concern about being anxious or angry, the therapist can ask whether they know anyone who 'never has worries'. This is not to downplay their distress or the fact that the aim of therapy is to help them feel better but to make it clear that therapy can't stop them from having worries or ever feeling angry or sad. Nor would it be right to do so. Adversities are part of life and there are times when it is appropriate to feel angry or sad (Trower et al. 2015).

In REBT the aim is to replace self-defeating evaluations to elicit more helpful emotions. The idea is that emotions fuel different kinds of behaviour and this is consistent with theories of emotion, which suggest that they play a key motivational role in human action (Damasio 2003). For example, if you are depressed then you may feel a sense of hopelessness and it may be difficult to deal with everyday challenges whereas sadness is unlikely to be as demotivating. In REBT a distinction is made between healthy versus unhealthy emotions (Trower et al. 2015). Most of us have experienced shameful moments and can imagine the crippling effects of trying to live with an overwhelming sense of shame. Unfortunately, talking about making these shifts between healthy and unhealthy emotions is a step too far for most people with intellectual disabilities. They find it difficult to label and talk about complex emotions like shame and embarrassment (Matheson and Jahoda 2005). This doesn't mean that people don't have a rich emotional life; rather, it requires a high level of receptive and expressive verbal ability to talk about your emotional life (Moore 2001). An important job the therapist has to do at the outset of therapy is to find a common language for talking about emotions and to do the groundwork by talking about different ways that feelings can be helpful and unhelpful to us. For example, feeling anxious about going to a new work placement can help someone to be prepared and alert when taking on new challenges. However, if someone becomes overanxious it can lead to panic and being unable to cope with the new demands or even result in them refusing to go in the first place.

A Shared Formulation

There are different approaches to producing a CBT formulation. At its heart, the idea of a formulation is to produce an account of people's difficulties using the CBT model. This account is then linked to a plan of work to address people's difficulties. More than this, an agreed formulation with the client helps to ensure there is a shared understanding of the person's difficulties and common cause when moving forward. Sometimes it can be useful to share the formulation with significant others in the client's life, to help them understand the client's difficulties. A better understanding can lead to a greater willingness to help the client, because it increases the support person's empathy. Other support workers might be very empathic but feel stuck and the formulation might give them new ideas about what they can do to help. However, the client needs to give their permission for their formulation to be shared with others.

One commonly used approach to CBT formulation is often referred to as the 'hot cross bun' (Greenberger and Padesky 1995), so called because it looks at the relationship between the four key interacting factors: Physiology, Behaviour, Cognition and Affect. The hot cross bun can be used to explain Jean's anxiety in the restaurant, where her thoughts (Cognitions) about being stared at by the waiter resulted in her beginning to experience the symptoms of panic (Physiology). Consequently she tried to avoid eye contact (Behaviour), which only made her more conscious of her rising sense of panic and less able to pick up on evidence that contradicted her view of the situation (Label). As her panic increased her wish to get out of the restaurant grew. The relief (Affect) she felt when she left the restaurant only served to reinforce her belief that the threat she had faced was real (Cognition).

While this approach to formulation is helpful and allows the therapist to use the CBT model to explain people's difficulties, the focus is on the internal cognitive system. People's wider social context is only a consideration insofar as it acts as a trigger or feeds into this cognitive system. The drawback of the 'hot cross bun' approach is that it does not capture a more holistic understanding of the person and the meaning of their distress in the wider context of their lives.

Tarrier and Calam (2002) proposed that there is a need to take account of interpersonal and social factors when formulating psychological interventions for any client group. He suggested that the decision about other social and interpersonal factors to include in formulations should draw on the evidence about psychosocial factors known to have an impact on people's emotional well-being. For example, poverty, social isolation, lack of emotional support, little meaningful activity and victimisation are all known to have a negative impact on people's mental health. All of these factors are germane to the lives of people with intellectual disabilities. Moreover, these are not only important factors to consider as part of a formulation; they may also play a crucial role in a CBT intervention.

The notion of taking a more holistic and systemic tack fits with the 5 Ps approach to formulation (Ingham et al. 2008). The 5 Ps are what is the *problem*; what made the person vulnerable to the problem or *predisposing factors*; why now and what triggered the problem or *precipitating factors*; what keeps the problem going or *perpetuating factors*; and what prevents the person's problems from getting worse or gives them strengths to build on in order to achieve and maintain a recovery or *protective factors*. Even though this approach isn't specifically a CBT-based model, it still offers a helpful way of formulating the client's difficulties in the wider context of their lives, including information that will help the client to achieve and maintain change. Of course, it's not only about the negatives; crucially it's also about finding out about how to build on people's strengths. This includes personal qualities, including people's skills and interests. However, people's strengths are not only internal, they also include the formal and informal supports and relationships that a person has. For example, people who face difficulties at work might gain solace from their fulfilling family life or their sporting success. Enjoying a range of achievements or having a number of valued social roles is thought to protect against depression (Linville 1987).

Dave Dagnan (2007) also offered a thoughtful account of the individual and contextual factors that should be taken into account when developing psychosocial formulations and interventions for people with intellectual disabilities. Rather than just setting out a list of individual or social factors that should be considered, he looked at the potential dynamic relationship between the individual and their environment. For example, does someone feel frustrated or somewhat hopeless when living as an adult within an overprotective environment? What is the impact of trying to manage on a small budget, with limited numeracy skills and only two hours of outreach support a week? Considering these dynamic factors highlights the value of multidisciplinary work and taking into account the work of health and social work colleagues and third sector social care providers (see Chap. 10). Other factors to take into account will be the management of long-term health conditions like epilepsy and chronic pain.

Stigma is another dynamic factor to be considered, even though there has been a tendency to view it as a static phenomenon or a form of negative life event. Being called names, left out or overprotected might all have a negative impact on an individual's self-perceptions or underlying self-schema, linked to low self-esteem and a lack of self-confidence. It follows that someone might internalise a negative, stigmatised view of self. However, this is only part of the story. While there may be some individuals who internalise a stigmatised view of self, the evidence suggests this is not a common occurrence (Jahoda and Markova 2004; Crabtree et al. 2010), or at least not in this straightforward fashion. Most people recognise that they have an intellectual disability but they do not necessarily think that it defines them as a person. In other words, people might talk about their difficulties with reading and writing or coping with aspects of everyday life like handling money and say this is due to having a disability. However, they are still likely to feel that they should be able to make their own decisions, deserve to be listened to and afforded the same respect and life opportunities as other people.

Goffman's (1963) book *Stigma: Notes on the Management of a Spoiled Identity* inspired a longitudinal study (Jahoda et al. 2010) in which we explored the lives of young people with clinically significant anxiety or depression at the stage of transition into adulthood. These young people were acutely aware of their stigmatised status but did not accept this identity. However, their struggles to manage their own identities were linked to the distress some of them experienced. One young man's attempt to seek acceptance from his peers at a local nightclub ended with an attempt to throw himself in front of a car after he was spat on by another youth. Perhaps more commonly, people simply avoid situations where they may experience discrimination or abuse. We often hear clients say they don't use public transport at times when children and young people are travelling to and from school.

Another of the participants in the ethnographic study of young people with significant problems of anxiety or depression lived at home with her mother. She was frustrated by the limited life opportunities that she had.

Many of the restrictions imposed on her, such as being prevented from using the cooker, were due to her mother's overprotectiveness. This left her feeling helpless and conflicted because she enjoyed a close and loving relationship with her mother. Thus, when exploring clients' experiences of stigma, the therapist needs to bear in mind that stigmatised treatment is not always imposed by distant others with cruel intentions.

An advantage of taking account of a broader range of social and psychological factors is that it offers a range of possible entry points for CBT with clients who may struggle with more abstract work concerning cognitions. For example, directing efforts at increasing a client's meaningful daytime activity could be tied into attempts to challenge depressive ideation and increase their confidence. There is also a B in CBT that incorporates behavioural approaches.

Tarrier (2006) helpfully suggested that a formulation could be described as a testable hypothesis or theory and that care should be taken to gather evidence allowing the hypothesis to be rejected as well as supported. This means that formulations need to be linked to a plan of what the therapist and client are going to work on together in sessions, and should include an agreed list of problems to be addressed and agreed ways of tackling them. If the plan doesn't work or circumstances change, then the formulation can be revised. Of course, clinically significant change measured by a self-report measure of clinical symptoms is one thing but knowing how this might translate into real-world change is another. For example, the goal for someone who has anger management problems might not only be to gain more control over their anger but to cope with social gatherings that he or she is currently excluded from due to their frequent aggression.

Having real-life therapeutic goals can help to make the time-limited nature of therapy explicit and means there has to be a discussion about what change is possible. In truth, not all of clients' problems will be solved by CBT. The idea to get across is that even small changes could make a real difference to someone or be the beginning of a process of change that they could continue. Once again, this will often mean moving beyond individual work, to consider other systemic factors and the support needed to make meaningful change. There would be little point working with someone to become less agoraphobic, only to find that they still rarely leave their house because they don't have anyone to go out with or have no access to transport.

One way of reaching agreement about a formulation is to produce a draft formulation booklet. The draft can be discussed with the client before it is finalised. When discussing the formulation, it can be made clear to the client that their views are important and that changes will be made to incorporate their views. The final agreed version can be given to the client. New technology means that a final copy of the formulation could be given to the client in a number of formats, including a short audio recording.

Jean—Formulation

The following section outlines a formulation developed for Jean. The aim was to present an accessible formulation that made sense to her and offered the basis for joint work together. The version that was discussed and shared with her is presented in the form of an accessible booklet (and can be found on the website www.toolsfortalking.wordpress.com). With Jean's agreement, her mum was also given a copy of the formulation.

Formulation Presented

Jean has had experience of being bullied in the past, being made to feel different and left out. She had a particularly hard time in her teenage years from children in her neighbourhood who used to call her names. So it is understandable that she is anxious about what other people think about her and worries about making mistakes. When she begins to feel panic she worries even more about what other people will think of her, believing that her racing heart and feeling hot and bothered means something terrible is going to happen. At these times she just wants to return to the safety of her own home.

Jean's anxiety and inability to cope with different social situations has been exacerbated by the loss of meaningful and regular activity since she left school, and she spends most of her time on her own in her bedroom. Having limited company and social support has also contributed to low mood and a sense of hopelessness about her situation. Understandably, Jean's mum's main concern has been to keep her safe and help her to avoid her becoming distressed. Thus, there seems to be something of a vicious circle that has contributed to Jean's growing level of distress. It could be explained in the following way:

Leaving school meant losing both friends and regular activity, leading to a loss of self-confidence. This has made her more anxious about going out, raising fears about how others would view her and increasing her tendency to look away from others when she begins to experience panic. Although she avoids eye contact to help her feel safer (safety behaviour), in reality it just makes things worse because her attention is turned inwards on to her feelings of panic. Being more aware of having a churning stomach and racing heart just makes her panic more! Due to her anxiety she has become more reluctant to leave the house and doesn't take advantage of the opportunities that she is afforded, making her feel down and hopeless. It also emphasises her reliance on her parents for her support, increasing her worry about what will happen in the future when her parents are no longer there to support her.

Positively, in terms of protective factors, Jean has a very supportive family. Moreover, she is an engaging and sociable individual who wants to develop more relationships with people of her own age and still loves going to the classes she attends and is surprisingly confident when playing roles in her drama group. Finally, she is motivated to engage in therapy and to play an active part in the process. Despite having very limited literacy skills she has completed the daily recording sheets she has been given and the other homework tasks that were agreed, with the help of her mum.

Working Together: The Way Forward

Firstly, a programme of graded exposure, with the aim of increasing Jean's routine activity, will be drawn up. This programme will consist of a gradual series of steps towards reducing her anxiety about going into public places. The first step will be to go to a quiet café near her home, supported by her mum. The next steps will be to go to slightly busier cafes. During these excursions, Jean will be encouraged to drop her safety behaviour and look around her, with the aim of reducing her fear of the threat posed by others. A series of gradual steps will lead to her final goal, meeting a friend for lunch.

The linked work in sessions will aim to (i) address her tendency to catastrophise about the physical symptoms of anxiety, including tackling her belief that these physical symptoms mean something terrible is going to happen, and (ii) tackle her negative self-evaluations linked to anxiety about how she is viewed by others.

Related work will also be carried out to boost her self-esteem, drawing attention to her strengths and her motivation to achieve change. Finally, help will be given to find new activities that offer Jean a chance to meet and build relationships with people of her own age group.

To allay mum's anxiety about therapy, the formulation and proposals for the therapeutic work will be carefully presented, in order to make it clear that therapy would involve very gradual steps with the aim of reducing Jean's distress. Otherwise, there is a risk that mum would withdraw Jean from therapy, as she relies on mum's support to travel to meet with the therapist. Very positively, when asked about her goals for therapy, Jean has said that she wants to increase her confidence and to meet more people of her own age. So the goals of therapy are in keeping with Jean's wishes.

Remember, the formulation is not written in tablets of stone. While the formulation should offer the basis for an agreed programme of joint work, this often changes over time as the sessions progress and unforeseen challenges arise or new issues come to the fore.

This first stage of CBT should include generic components of a good talking therapy, ensuring that the clients' concerns are listened to and offering suggestions for joint work together that instil hope. Sometimes this first stage of therapy, which gives the client an opportunity to tell someone about the nature of their difficulties and gain more understanding of their feelings, is all they may wish for.

> **Key Points**
> - In the first phase of therapy the client should, at least, develop a sense of the structure and purpose of sessions, if not an understanding of the CBT model itself.
> - The therapist, in turn, needs to develop an understanding of the client's interpersonal and communicative style.
> - Talking about emotive events may be a more effective way of helping clients to make sense of the CBT model, rather than reflecting in a more abstract way on thoughts and feelings.
> - The formulation process should take account of the wider context of the client's life and the dynamic relationship between the individual and their environment. CBT should not be used as a panacea for social disadvantage faced by people with intellectual disabilities.

References

Bruce, M., Collins, S., Langdon, P., Powlitch, S., & Reynolds, S. (2010). Does training improve understanding of core concepts in cognitive behaviour therapy by people with intellectual disabilities? A randomized experiment. *British Journal of Clinical Psychology, 49*, 1–13.

Crabtree, J. W., Haslam, S. A., Postmes, T., & Haslam, C. (2010). Mental health support groups, stigma, and self-esteem: Positive and negative implications of social identification. *Journal of Social Issues, 66*(3), 553–569.

Cuthill, F. M., Espie, C. A., & Cooper, S.-A. (2003). Development and psychometric properties of the Glasgow depression scale for people with a learning disability. *British Journal of Psychiatry, 182*, 347–353.

Dagnan, D. (2007). Psychosocial interventions for people with intellectual disabilities and mental ill-health. *Current Opinion in Psychiatry, 20*, 456–460.

Dagnan, D., & Chadwick, P. (1997). Cognitive-behaviour therapy for people with learning disabilities: Assessment and intervention. In B. Stenfert Kroese, D. Dagnan, & E. Lumidis (Eds.), *Cognitive behaviour therapy for people with learning disabilities* (pp. (162–(181). London: Routledge.

Damasio, A. (2003). Feelings of emotion and the self. *Annals of the New York Academy of Science, 1001*, 253–261.

Goffman, E. (1963). *Stigma: Notes on the management of a spoiled identity*. Englewood Cliffs: Prentice Hall.

Greenberger, D., & Padesky, C. A. (1995). *Mind over mood: A cognitive therapy treatment manual for clients*. New York: Guilford Press.

Hebblethwaite, A., Jahoda, A., & Dagnan, D. (2011). Talking about real life events: An investigation of the ability of people with intellectual disabilities to make links between their beliefs and emotions within dialogue. *Journal of Applied Research in Intellectual Disability, 24*, 543–553.

Ingham, B., Clark, L., & James, I. A. (2008). Biopsychosocial case formulation for people with intellectual disabilities and mental health problems: A pilot study of a training workshop for direct care staff. *The British Journal of Developmental Disabilities, 54*(1), 41–54.

Jahoda, A., & Markova, I. (2004). Coping with social stigma: People with intellectual disabilities moving from institutions and the family home. *Journal of Intellectual Disability Research, 48*(8), 719–729.

Jahoda, A., Wilson, A., Stalker, K., & Cairney, A. (2010). Living with stigma and the self-perceptions of people with mild intellectual disabilities. *Journal of Social Issues, 66*(3), 521–534.

Kirk, J. D., Jahoda, A., & Pert, C. (2008). Beliefs about aggression and submissiveness: A comparison of aggressive and nonaggressive individuals with mild intellectual disability. *Journal of Mental Health and Intellectual Disability, 1*, 91–204.

Linville, P. W. (1987). Self-complexity as a cognitive buffer against stress-related illness and depression. *Journal of Personality and Social Psychology, 52*, 663–676.

Matheson, E., & Jahoda, A. (2005). Emotional understanding in aggressive and non-aggressive individuals with mild and moderate mental retardation. *American Journal on Mental Retardation, 110*, 57–67.

Moore, D. (2001). Reassessing emotion recognition performance in people with mental retardation: A review. *American Journal on Mental Retardation, 106*, 481–502.

McRitchie, R., McKenzie, K., Quayle, E., Harlin, M., & Neumann, K. (2013). How adults with an intellectual disability experience bereavement and grief: A qualitative exploration. *Death Studies, 38*, 1–7.

Tarrier, N., & Calam, R. (2002). New developments in cognitive-behavioural case formulation. Epidemiological, systemic and social context: An integrative approach. *Cognitive and Behavioural Psychotherapy, 30*, 311–328.

Tarrier, N. (2006). An introduction to case formulation and its challenges. In N. Tarrier & J. Johnson (Eds.), *Case formulation in cognitive behaviour therapy: The treatment of complex and challenging cases* (pp. 1–11). London: Routledge.

Trower, P., Jones, J., & Dryden, W. (2015). *Cognitive-behavioural counselling in action* (3rd ed.). London: Sage.

Westbrook, D., Mueller, M., Kennerley, H., & McManus, F. (2010). Common problems in therapy. In M. Mueller, H. Kennerley, F. McManus, & D. Westbrook (Eds.), *The Oxford guide to surviving as a CBT therapist*. Oxford: Oxford University Press.

6

Therapeutic Change

In this chapter, we deal with the next stage of therapy, where the aim is to work towards therapeutic change and finish therapy. The formulation provides a shared focus for the therapist's and client's endeavours. This includes behavioural tasks alongside cognitive work about how the clients think, feel and how they see themselves and others. Although these elements of the CBT model are interlinked we will deal with each therapeutic component in turn, before considering the end of therapy. Helping clients to achieve change is not simply about pure technique, it can also be seen as an art. Developing key competencies to deliver a therapy like CBT, accompanied by the appropriate values, is usually thought to be sufficient to become a good therapist, but this does not take account of the creative process of therapy.

In Eric Kandel's (2012) extraordinary book *The Age of Insight*, he explores the relationships between Freud's theory of psychological life, including unconscious processes, and the groundbreaking expressionist art emerging in Austria at the time. He links Freud's grasp of the unconscious to the daring developments of artists like Schiele, Klimt and Kokoshka, who tried to engage the viewer emotionally. Kandel goes on to consider these developments in light of current neuroscience and the nature of the 'social brain'. He draws parallels between the creative process of art and storytelling, and the ability of the visual artist to provide the viewer with a different view of the world:

> Stories, like works of visual art, are highly organized models of reality that narrator and listener alike can repeat and turn over in their own minds, examining relations between characters acting in different social and environmental settings. Storytelling is a low-risk way of solving survival problems in the imagination. It is also a source of information. Along with the size of the human brain, language and storytelling enable us to model our world uniquely and to communicate these models to others. (p. 393)

Consistent with the CBT model, Kandel talks about the creative process in the human brain being cognitive, emotional and empathic. Using CBT to achieve change is about helping clients find new insights into ways of thinking and behaving that reduces their distress. Being creative does not necessarily mean being complicated, just the opposite. The aim is to make CBT meaningful and emotionally engaging for clients. Most therapists we know who use CBT with people who have an intellectual disability are constantly striving to bring the therapy to life for those they are working with. Being creative is entirely consistent with a rigorous approach to therapy and a strength, not something to apologise about. For example, pictures might help a client who struggles to find the right words to talk about their worries. Another client may be confused by the therapist's attempt to explain the impact of overgeneralising from limited evidence. One possibility might be to use the example of a character from a TV programme the client is a fan of, who is always jumping to conclusions. Bear in mind this creative aspect of therapy as we look at what might be different in helping people who have intellectual disabilities work towards change when using CBT.

Picture drawn by a client with an intellectual disability who felt very depressed.

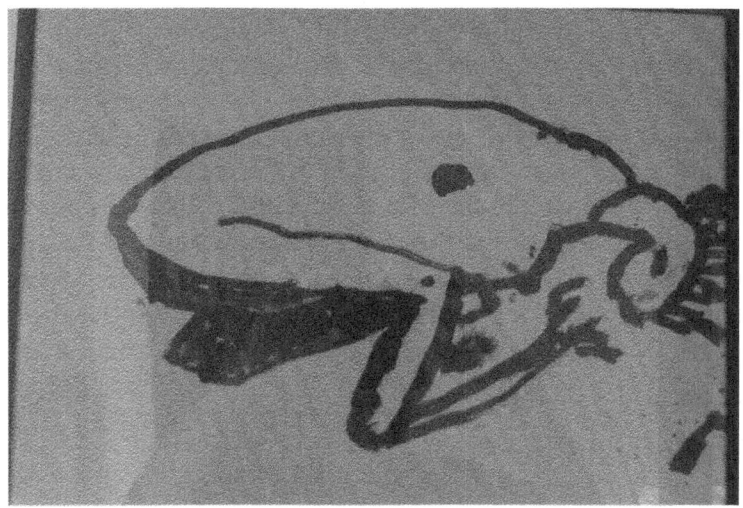

A Continuing Need for Structure

This creative aspect of therapy is framed by a continuing structure and sense of purpose, and setting an agenda plays a crucial part in this. Agendas will tend to follow a similar pattern across sessions. A starting point might be to recap briefly on what happened in the previous session, to try and ensure continuity. This is likely to be followed by an attempt to catch up with what has happened since the last session (including a review of any mood or self-report diaries that have been kept), then homework tasks might be reviewed. This would lead into the main work to be carried out in the session, before taking time to reflect on what has been covered and confirming the date and time for the next meeting. Of course, when setting an agenda, you need to make sure that you are giving priority to pressing issues clients want to talk about. An advantage of having an agenda is that it helps to keep the therapist and client on track, as some clients may perseverate about particular issues or have shifting preoccupations from week to week.

Despite the best efforts of the therapist, the therapy session can still become chaotic at times. It might reflect the real difficulties a client is facing and their sense of powerlessness to control events in their lives. Sometimes clients may just lack more tangible support. For example, we have worked with people who have brought bills or official letters to sessions because they couldn't read them or did not know what to do and who had no one else to turn to for help. Of course, sessions might feel out of control because the client becomes confused about the purpose of therapy or the therapist has their own preoccupations and isn't paying proper attention to where the client wants to go. Sometimes opportunities arise out of chaos, revealing what's emotionally salient for the client and giving the therapist openings to bring CBT into relevant discussions.

Behavioural Change

Seeking to understand how people with an intellectual disability interpret and make sense of their position in the world may also be revealed by their actions. Helping clients to change what they do or how they cope can be explicitly linked to their self and interpersonal perceptions. For example, a therapist might work with a client who has anger problems to help them respond less aggressively in situations of interpersonal conflict. The client's improvement might reasonably be attributed to greater self-control. However, behaving differently will also result in less conflict and change how other people respond to them. It would seem to be a rather one-dimensional view to assume that people with intellectual disabilities only learn to exert greater self-control in a mechanistic fashion and lack agency or fail to attach meaning to their actions or the reactions of others. A client could feel good about being more in control and developing better relationships with other people. Behavioural approaches are a core aspect of CBT with people who have intellectual disabilities, but the 'self' who is learning to change or regulate their behaviour needs to be acknowledged (Jahoda et al. 2001).

We talked in the last chapter about the advantages of setting agreed goals to work towards, which are meaningful to clients. Behavioural techniques like self-regulation, graded exposure, scheduled activities and problem solving all have the advantage of being more concrete with observable outcomes, and can be easier for clients to grasp and to play an active role in. These approaches are about real-world change, which extend beyond the therapy session. However, there can be both motivational and practical barriers to completing behavioural plans. Clients may lack the agency or control in their lives to plan and carry through with actions. They can also face significant organisational barriers, such as insufficient or inflexible support arrangements (see also Chaps. 3, 4 and 5). There is no point in scheduling a positive event like going swimming if the client needs someone to accompany them but their support worker can't or won't swim.

If clients need support to carry out activities between sessions, then these activities are likely to need careful thought and planning if they are to happen. This includes looking at potential barriers and what is going to be helpful. Plans might include *where*, *when* and *with whom* an activity will happen. This could mean enlisting the support of a significant other in the person's life, which might be a support worker, family member, partner or friend. When someone else is involved they need to know why an activity is being planned and the therapist should check if the support person is in agreement. Otherwise, the support person may lack the motivation to help, or even prove to be obstructive if they think it is a bad idea. If the therapist knows from their early sessions that the client is likely to need support with behavioural plans, then the best way of managing it would be to involve the support person from the beginning. This means that the therapist can negotiate a plan that both the client and the support person are willing to sign up to.

In the UK, where therapists often work as part of a team of professionals supporting people with intellectual disabilities, it is sometimes possible to enlist the help of colleagues like community nurses or other outreach workers, to support people carry out homework tasks. On occasion, it might be a good idea for the therapist to support the client. For example, if a client is socially anxious a key part of the intervention might be a programme of graded exposure, to allow them go out into public places again. It might reach a stage when there is little point in the therapist continuing to talk about the problem when none of the ideas are being translated into steps towards real change. One way forward might be for the therapist to accompany the client to a nearby café or shopping centre, as part of their session. There can also be occasions where the therapist believes that it is important for them to do the behavioural work with the clients directly, whether or not other support is available. It would be wrong for therapists to believe that the behavioural components of the intervention are beneath them and should always be delegated to less qualified colleagues. Working in vivo not only offers therapists a chance to help clients put therapy into practice, it also helps to build rapport with the client and to develop an understanding of how they think and feel when facing challenges and provides insight into the practical barriers to achieving change.

Clients' own motivation is essential for change, and time should be taken to review their progress in carrying through behavioural plans during therapy sessions. The therapist should talk about what works, as well as identify the barriers to progress. Again, make sure the client is involved in recording their progress with homework tasks. Remember, it is more important to engage the client in the process, rather than having a complicated recording sheet. We have already talked about simple and effective ideas such as using simple tick box charts or asking the support person or client to take a photograph of what they do, using their phone or a camera.

The therapist should keep in mind that behavioural work is embedded in the client's *cognitive behavioural* formulation. Therefore, helping them to change their behaviour should tie in with efforts to help people reflect on their underlying beliefs about self and the world. For example, a client might have started therapy with the view 'don't try new things because you'll get it wrong then everyone will think you're stupid and it'll make you feel terrible'. Reflecting on their success in starting a new college course might lead to a new way of thinking that 'it's good to give things a try, everyone has to start somewhere'. Or maybe there will be a more modest shift in the client's views and they will be less likely to believe that trying something new will end in disaster. When clients successfully complete agreed tasks it offers an opportunity for increasing their self-confidence and encouraging more helpful ways of thinking about challenges they face.

Even when clients do successfully carry through with planned activities, sometimes they still fail to give themselves credit for their achievements. Such a reaction is perhaps unsurprising if one of their core problems is a negative view of self or an external locus of control. This is one of the reasons why behavioural work alone may not be sufficient to produce meaningful change.

Establishing a Therapeutic Dialogue

Listening properly to what clients say can be more challenging when people have communicative and cognitive difficulties. There is good guidance available to help therapists to communicate effectively. Lindsay et al. (2013) suggest that therapists should use short sentences, straightforward language and repetition to help ensure that they are understood. However, therapeutic dialogue is just that, more than the individual contributions of the therapist and the client. There can be a risk that if the therapist becomes too self-conscious about adjusting or simplifying their language the interaction will become stilted. In a study investigating therapeutic dialogue between therapists and clients with intellectual disabilities (Jahoda et al. 2009), we found that they did manage to establish collaborative dialogues in CBT sessions. The novel form of analysis used in that study was developed to investigate the flow and balance of dialogue between two individuals, coding how one communicative partner's turn linked to the other person's contribution (Linell et al. 1988). Perhaps unsurprisingly, the therapists asked most of the questions but the clients appeared to be actively engaged in the discussions and their answers usually helped to keep the topic of conversation alive. It appeared that the therapists' approach was not just about simplifying their communication to make it more accessible but that they were scaffolding the conversation to help the participants to engage with the process.

The dialogues we recorded between the therapists and clients with intellectual disabilities did not resemble typical case examples given in CBT textbooks, where elegant questioning appears to elicit thoughtful reflection from the clients. The therapists and clients were often ungrammatical, in the sense that what they said did not lend itself easily to a comprehensible written account. Sometimes the therapists' ums and errs and rather complicated questions were painful to read. So the successful dialogues could not just be explained by the use of simple, clear language.

Building a dialogue was also about the therapists' broader approach to the conversation, including taking an interest in what the client said and finding ways that allowed the client to talk about matters that are important to them.

Trying to communicate in a more accessible fashion or working to compensate for clients' cognitive difficulties is not quite the same as trying to build a collaborative therapeutic relationship. Collaborative working means allowing or assisting clients to find their voice and to play an active role in sessions. Key to this is making it clear to clients, who may not always be used to putting forward their point of view, that they have something important to say. This fits with Vygotsky's ideas about supporting another person's engagement in activity; it is about motivating and interesting them in the task, rather than just making it straightforward to carry out.

The following is a piece of dialogue between a therapist (T) and a client (C), who were part of our study examining communication in CBT with people who have intellectual disabilities (Jahoda et al. 2009). The client had visual impairments and he was talking about the unease he felt when his support staff were quiet.

> *T*: Superb. So you were saying that you thought that if people were quiet with you, they would think you were doing something wrong, yeah?
> *C*: Yep. Yes.
> *T*: Basically you were thinking that …
> *C*: I've done something wrong.
> *T*: You've done something wrong.
> *C*: Mm hmm. Yep.
> *T*: And when you start thinking that, how do you start feeling?
> *C*: Bad. Guilty.
> *T*: Mm hmm. Mm hmm. Worried?
> *T*: Yep.
> *T*: OK. OK.
> *C*: Because I end up going is there something wrong? Have I said something that I shouldn't have said? [T: Mm hmm] But sometimes I wonder if they're just saying that [T: Mm hmm] for the sake of saying it. Or do they mean it?
> *T*: OK. OK. (Jahoda and Markova, I. 2004)

Working with Thoughts and Feelings (Bottom Up and Top Down)

Not only will the therapist and client have an agreed formulation and goals for therapy by this stage but there should also be completed self-monitoring sheets or, at the very least, a record of recent salient events in the client's life. This means that there should be a direction and material to work on for the cognitive-emotional part of therapy.

Socratic Questioning In most accounts of CBT, the core technique for working with clients' cognitions is the Socratic method (Lindsay et al. 2015). This is a way of asking clients questions that helps them to become more aware of the assumptions underpinning their thoughts and behaviour. It fits with the notion that clients are being asked to become lay scientists in therapy, testing out how their thoughts, behaviour and physiological symptoms are linked to their emotional well-being. The challenge, when working with people who have an intellectual disability, is to avoid the Socratic approach becoming a confusing intellectual exercise that they struggle to engage with. The last thing people with emotional problems need is a therapeutic technique which heightens their anxiety, sense of inadequacy or frustration.

Let's look at the example of a therapist who wants to explore a client's view that a support worker was 'ignoring' him and is a 'nasty' person because she arrived at his home ten minutes later than expected. A Socratic question might be, 'What makes you think that the support worker was ignoring you?' This might prove to be a very helpful starting point with some clients but for others it might lead straight back to their original conclusion, 'because they're not nice, they should be there on time'.

An alternative approach is to try to scaffold the question. A starting point might be to try and establish a fuller picture: 'tell me more about what happened this morning?' This question might lead onto a discussion about the regular pattern of help that the support worker offers to different people in the block of flats. Building on this background information could also help the client to consider other possible reasons or motivations for the worker behaving the way she did. Even at this stage, asking the client directly about their reason for thinking the staff member had been ignoring him may not prove fruitful. However, suggesting an alternative reason based on the information the client has provided might prove more successful. 'Do you think that the worker was ignoring you or do you think that she was just busy working with your neighbour?' Any alternatives put forward by the therapists need to be plausible and make sense to the client, built on an understanding of the individual and their circumstances.

A heightened sensitivity to rejection might be linked to the client's sense of ill treatment and feelings of humiliation or anger. Opening up the possibility of seeing events in a different way may help to shift a client's negative evaluations. Even if the participant lacks literacy skills, writing or drawing out the client's thoughts and responses to the event on a large piece of paper, as described in the previous chapter, can help to make the process more accessible. Moreover, the clients can take the sheets (or photos of the sheets) away with them at the end of the session, reinforcing the fact that the work has been completed jointly.

In general adult mental health, CBT therapists have expert knowledge of the model (metacompetence) and use this knowledge to guide the therapeutic dialogue in a creative manner. So it should not be considered a problem if people with intellectual disabilities require more scaffolding to allow them to consider different perspectives.

Role Play The value of using role play was introduced in the last chapter. One of the advantages of role play is that the person is acting out different ways of dealing with an event, so the therapist is able to help the client to reflect on their thoughts and actions as the scenario unfolds.

In terms of working towards change, role play offers the chance to take a situation through to its conclusion and to consider the cycle of difficulties that people might find themselves caught in. Let us say that a therapist and a client called John role-play a recent incident of conflict, with the therapist playing the neighbour John has fallen out with. During the role play John ends up saying that he would get involved in a fight with his neighbour, leading to a discussion about the consequences for John and how he is viewed and treated by others. John might say that other people will become afraid of him and start to avoid him, feeding into his view (inference) that others ignore him, which he thinks (evaluation) is unfair. So John ends up thinking 'I am the one who is being treated badly, I am a victim'. The therapist could then draw out this cycle of conflict and discuss what would happen if John acted differently, including how he would end up seeing himself. Then they could act out this different sequence of events.

The role play might also reveal the subtly different feelings that John might find it hard to put into words. John might say he ends up feeling really distressed when he gets angry and loses control, while at the same time believing that anger is an effective way of making others listen to him. To address this apparent contradiction, the therapist and John could reframe their work from achieving greater self-control in anger-provoking situations to being about 'becoming the boss' and being the one who 'keeps control'.

Role play or 'doing some acting' can be used to address different difficulties that the client wishes to discuss or that are recorded in the diary they bring with them. Importantly, the role plays can also be linked to homework tasks, helping to generalise the use of different evaluations in the client's everyday life. Of course, role play will not suit everyone and for some people the use of drawings, photographs, video and other materials might be alternative ways of promoting engagement with therapeutic work.

Whatever materials the therapist uses, care needs to be taken to ensure that any alternative inferences or evaluations they put forward are meaningful to the client. Just suggesting a different way of thinking isn't enough. We all have the experience of wishing things were different or recognising that our views are irrational but it making no difference to how we actually feel. *I know there's no point in worrying about that but …*

It's crucial for therapists to check if clients think their suggestions are helpful. Asking clients to rate how much they believe a particular thought or view is true for them is one way of finding out if they agree with a suggestion that has been made and charting how views change. For example, one of the authors has a beautiful set of small weighing scales. These scales look as if they are used to measure out small quantities of mind-altering substances rather than psychological therapies! The scales can be used in therapy to weigh up the pros and cons of different thoughts that have been generated, by adding or taking away weights. Evidence of positive change can be gauged by the increasing weight given to alternative thoughts that are less distressing.

Of course, the way people interpret events will not always be consistent or one dimensional. Clients with anger problems may sometimes find someone's actions infuriating and at other times less aggravating. They may feel angry and frustrated, angry and sad or angry and uptight. These inconsistencies and variations can be helpful, insofar as they demonstrate that different ways of viewing similar events lead to different feelings. We are not tied to one view of the world or one set of feelings. Moreover, there may also be times when people have coped with difficult events in an effective way. Gaining insight into effective solutions produced by clients themselves can be immensely useful to therapists. CBT therapy is also about building on a client's strengths, as someone who acts on and shapes their world in a positive way, rather than just getting them to reflect on their difficulties.

Top-Down Approaches and Behavioural Experiments

When Baron-Cohen carried out his early studies into theory of mind in autism (Baron-Cohen 1992), he often used people with Down syndrome as one of his control groups. One of these naturalistic experiments used the game where you have a coin hidden in one of your hands behind your back. You then bring both hands forward with your fists closed and ask the other person to guess which hand the coin is in. Three groups took part in his experiment: individuals with autism, typically developing youngsters and young people with Down syndrome. The young people with autism didn't prove to be terribly good at the task, as a lack of theory of mind meant that they found it difficult to second-guess their opponent and sometimes even failed to hide the coin. The typically developing young people engaged in quite a sophisticated process of trying to second-guess their opponent and shifting the coin between their hands. Whilst, on the whole, the young people with Down syndrome didn't do so well on the task, a number used the most sophisticated strategy of all: they hid the coin in one of their pockets!

There tends to be an assumption that to simplify a therapy like CBT for people with an intellectual disability means breaking it down into smaller components, as if you need to grasp the constituent parts in order to build up an understanding of the whole. This follows the same logic as breaking down a new skill into different tasks, in order to make the learning easier. So the first step in learning how to make a sandwich might just involve adding the fillings onto pieces of buttered bread using a technique called backward chaining. However, when dealing with socio-emotional issues, people can sometimes find it easier to understand the 'whole thing' or the 'gestalt'. Like the young people with Down syndrome, they get the point of the game, even if some of the complexities evade them.

For example, a therapist might become aware that a client like John who has anger management problems, described above, has a heightened view of threat from others, believing that they tend to put him down or treat him badly. Consequently, John avoids speaking to support staff who work with him and those living in neighbouring flats. Sadly, this only has the effect of fuelling his suspicions and making him feel that others are avoiding him. To break this cycle, the therapist needn't explain the A-B-C model to the client but instead might negotiate with the client to try the simple strategy of saying 'hello' to staff and other tenants, and to feel he is able to take 'control' in social situations. There could be other work in therapy sessions to reflect on the success of the strategy and its impact on the client's self and interpersonal perceptions but it does not necessarily rely on an in-depth discussion of A-B-C links.

The Way You Think

As we highlighted in the previous chapter, it's not just about how clients interpret events or judge themselves and other people that matter, it's also their thinking style. Being rigid or having a tendency to generalise from limited information can be maladaptive ways of dealing with the world. Even ordinary events, like being criticised for being untidy, might feel devastating or catastrophic: 'they must think I'm a bad person' or 'they're always picking on me and trying to put me down'. These types of errors not only lead clients to misinterpret events but they also help to guide and restrict their actions.

If clients are too quick to jump to a conclusion (or evaluation), then work also needs to be done to make them aware of their evaluative style. For example, when the therapist is talking to someone who is suffering from social anxiety problems the therapist might want to check if the client is always 'quick to think that they're making a fool of themselves' in public. Making these thinking styles more conscious is a starting point for negotiating more helpful approaches that clients can try out. For example, if someone is quick to catastrophise about making a fool of themselves in public then the therapist might ask 'what's the worst thing that could happen?' More often than not, the worst thing hasn't ever happened, allowing the therapist to go on to talk about advantages of using more evidence on which to base interpretations of events. Another potential approach the therapist might use is to draw up a list of situations where clients' first impressions had been wrong and to review the consequences.

Of course, jumping to a conclusion is not just a thinking style. Clients' approaches to events are also based on feelings they have about the world, themselves and their relationships with others. Knowing that 'the worst thing hasn't happened' may or may not help a client feel less anxious but the discussion with the therapist should be broader. It needs to be about what it *feels* like to know 'the worst has never happened' and to work out ways of building clients' confidence, making them less prone to catastrophising about being in social situations.

There is a risk that taking this approach can make the therapist a hostage to fortune because sometimes the worst can and does happen. One of us worked with a client who expressed a fear of becoming ill and drawing attention to herself when she became anxious. Then on one occasion she was physically sick when she visited a busy town centre because of her overwhelming level of anxiety. Fortunately, workers from a local shop were sympathetic and kind, and the client managed to cope with the situation well and she managed to complete her errand before returning home. Rather than being a setback, this proved to be a positive turning point in therapy as she did not feel that she had lost control and appreciated the help she received. A key component of the therapeutic work was to reinforce her sense of self as someone who had shown remarkable strength to deal with the considerable challenges in her life.

Whilst adapted CBT approaches may prove helpful, the question remains as to what should be done when clients' particular thinking styles are a hard-wired aspect of their developmental difficulty. For example, people with autism often have a rather rigid and literal thinking style, which could be thought of as fitting with the maladaptive patterns described in CBT theory (e.g. black and white, or either-or, thinking). It is interesting there is evidence that CBT has been successfully adapted for people with autism. Most of this work has been with those who have high-functioning autism or Asperger syndrome, who don't have an intellectual disability (Spain et al. 2014), and has largely focused on anxiety, the most commonly occurring emotional difficulty they face. Interestingly, a number of the suggested adaptations for people with autism overlap with those already suggested for those with intellectual disabilities. These adaptations aim to address problems with emotional understanding and perspective taking. They include the use of role play and visual aids to help make the ideas more concrete and to promote more adaptive ways of thinking and new coping strategies. Another interesting suggestion, when working with young people with autism, is to make positive use of their special interests, or their tendency to be passionate about certain characters or topics. For example, someone might have a passion for a film or television character like Dr Who. The character could then be used when giving examples of different ways of thinking and coping, helping to increase the person's engagement in therapy and galvanise their motivation to change.

It is likely that some people with intellectual disabilities who are referred for CBT will also be on the autistic spectrum. For these individuals, it is necessary to take account of the different ways that they might process events in the world. However, care has to be taken to avoid thinking that these individuals' emotional difficulties can always be explained by dint of having autism. Being socially marginalised, bullied or having limited meaningful activity has the same negative impact on those who have autism as on others. Moreover, those who have autism may have similar concerns to other people. I recall supervising a trainee who was working with a young man with mild intellectual disabilities and autism who presented with considerable anxiety and tearfulness. After an exhaustive assessment, concerning his adjustment to leaving school, we realised that too great a focus had been placed on his autism and key questions about the nature of his worries had not been addressed. So a general anxiety assessment, including a section with a series of questions about typical worries, was completed with him. It emerged that the recent illness of a relative had triggered considerable worries about his mother's health and anxiety about who would be there to support him when his mother died. Dealing directly with these concerns was highly effective for this young man.

Perceptions of Self and Working with Stigma

People's struggles with stigma are not just internal; they are about dealing with real stigmatised treatment that they face in everyday life. As stated previously, this might be about dealing with bullying or hate crime, which in turn might result in people avoiding particular social situations or locations.

CBT therapists work with the distress caused by clients' struggles with stigma by helping to change negative perceptions of self. The therapeutic aim is to try and promote a more positive identity and help clients find ways of dealing with stigma. In fact, people with intellectual disabilities themselves offer important insights into how to achieve these goals and research has shown that many people remain remarkably resilient in the face of stigma and refuse to be defined by their intellectual disability (Jahoda and Markova 2004). This does not necessarily mean that they wish to dissociate themselves from other people with an intellectual disability or deny having intellectual disabilities; they simply do not believe that they are less worthy as persons. However, even if they do not internalise a negative view of self, they might be hurt by the fact that others do not accept them or look down on them. Most clients will have a sense of what is fair and reasonable treatment, born out of an awareness of the wider social world of which they are a part and their strengths as well as weaknesses. Different approaches might be taken by the CBT therapist, depending on the nature of the clients' distress caused by the stigmatised treatment they face.

If clients have come to view themselves negatively due to other people's discriminatory views, then a focus for therapeutic work might be to explore whether their evaluations of self should be shaped by other people's prejudices. Straightforward techniques, such as drawing up a list of the clients' strengths and discussing what these tell the client about the kind of person they are, can be used to reinforce a positive sense of self. This might include asking the client to do some detective work of their own, and find out from significant others in their lives what they like about them and see as their strengths. Sometimes the therapist may think it best to assist the client with their detective work, as it could be counterproductive if some people were unkind.

Stigmatised treatment can have a corrosive effect on a client's sense of social self-efficacy. They might feel that they have no control over how they are perceived by others and feel hurt and rather hopeless about this, even if they know it is unjust. One way of tackling this sense of hopelessness might be to work on a life story book, emphasising the client's strengths and how they have coped with and overcome challenges. The advantage of life story work is that you end up with a book that the client can keep and continue to use, providing a positive sense of who they are. This does not mean ignoring the difficulties they have or the challenges that they face. Indeed, part of this process is to help them understand that the feelings they have about discrimination and rejection are normal and quite understandable. The emphasis should be on how they have managed to cope. Writing a letter to those who have bullied them or mistreated them in the past has a similar rationale, acknowledging the impact of their experience but aiming to overcome a sense of helplessness or shame they have been left with.

Robert Edgerton's (1967) book, *The Cloak of Competence,* describes his classic ethnographic study of a group of people with mild intellectual disabilities who were discharged from a large institution in California in the USA in the 1960s. As described in Chap. 2, he followed up these participants over a number of years to see how they fared. One of the challenges they faced was the stigma associated with having intellectual disabilities and having lived in long-stay institutions. What a number of these individuals did was to go out and buy old family photograph albums from second-hand shops and pass them off as their own. In order to have a future they needed to have a past.

Working with clients' identities is complicated and sometimes they can behave in ways that are paradoxical. I recall one woman with significant anxiety-related difficulties who dressed very flamboyantly, in keeping with her long-standing love of punk music. She also had a variety of facial piercings. She was so socially anxious that she would sit in cafes facing the wall to avoid eye contact with others. Of course, it would have been completely unhelpful to ask this woman to look round in the expectation that others would not stare at her or judge her. Equally, it would have been farcical to ignore her flamboyant appearance and lifestyle. Hence, we talked openly about her dress sense and appearance and her bravery to be her 'own person' with her 'own look'. We also considered what people who 'know her well' thought about her compared to those who met her for the first time. The worker who accompanied her to some of the sessions was very positive about her and spoke about what an engaging, gentle and thoughtful person she was. Tackling her appearance head on allowed us to work on gradually increasing her social activities and to reflect on the relationships she developed with others who got to know her, rather than judging her by her appearance. This tack also allowed us to address her depressed affect, linked to her loneliness, which was born out of fear of rejection by others.

Of course, it would be mistaken to think that it is only stigma relating to clients' intellectual disability that might arise. It's worth bearing in mind that people might struggle to be accepted in other ways; for example, if they wish to adopt a transsexual lifestyle and to cross-dress. Subtle skills and insights may be required to adopt such an identity successfully, which people with an intellectual disability might find difficult. The therapist may not be the best person to advise on an issue like that but they should be proactive in trying to get the client the help they need.

Real Changes

Dealing with stigma also highlights the need to work with the whole person and the multidisciplinary context when using CBT with people who have intellectual disabilities. If the aim is to build a client's confidence or self-esteem then it might also be about finding them social roles and relationships that provide them with something to feel proud or confident about.

> [S]ocial identities serve to structure (and restructure) people's perception and behaviour: their values, norms and goals; their orientations, relationships and interactions; what they think, what they do, and what they achieve. (Haslam 2014, p. 4)

Thus the therapist, alongside the client, might seek the assistance of social care colleagues to help someone find work or a volunteer role or to join a dance or music group. Having a broader range of social roles and activities of this nature also helps people to sustain well-being. We know that if we have a bad experience or feel demoralised by something that happens at work, it is important to have other aspects of life to fall back on that give us a sense of purpose or meaning.

From a social interactionist perspective, if a client is going to benefit from presenting a new, more confident face to the world, then they need others to acknowledge the difference (Jahoda et al. 2010). Symbolic interactionist theories of the self tell us that one of the ways we learn about ourselves is through others' behaviour towards us. Sometimes people with intellectual disabilities might not be taken seriously enough to get the recognition they want and deserve for the changes they are making. In these circumstances it might be appropriate for the therapist to ask if they can also work with significant others in the clients' lives, to try to shift their perceptions and responses. It is also worth reiterating that a good therapeutic relationship can have an important impact, in its own right—if the therapist listens to the client and takes their views seriously. Being listened to and having their views taken seriously might help to encourage a client's positive sense of self and agency.

Sometimes clients will reject an intellectual disability identity and will wish to distance themselves from other people with an intellectual disability (Haslam 2014). The therapist needs to respect this position. There will be some clients who are terribly isolated because even though they reject the identity of having an intellectual disability, they still struggle to achieve acceptance from others. In these instances, it is important to try to work alongside social care colleagues to ensure that support is provided in a sensitive fashion to help build the social connections essential for their well-being.

Finally, some individuals who are accepting of their label of having an intellectual disability may benefit in joining a self-advocacy or pressure group that works to promote more positive public attitudes. Consciousness raising and developing a positive sense of identity from being part of a mutually supportive group can have real therapeutic value.

Let's now return to Jean who we developed a formulation for in Chap. 5, and consider how we work with her to achieve therapeutic change.

Working with Jean (Continued from Chap. 5)
The agreed aims for Jean were to help her to become (i) more confident and learn that she could cope with getting out and about, with the ultimate goal of meeting up with a friend in the town centre for a coffee, and (ii) to look up rather than avoiding eye contact for fear that other people would stare at her. In turn, this was linked to her focus on internal physiological symptoms of panic and catastrophising about them. So the final aim was to (iii) help Jean become less distressed by the physiological symptoms of anxiety that she experienced.

This was all discussed in straightforward terms with Jean: 'To learn that you are okay and can cope when you go out to busier places means giving it a try. If you manage to stay out somewhere long enough you'll begin to calm down.' A big motivation for Jean was that she wanted to get to know more people and get back in touch with old friends.

In psychological terms, a number of steps were taken to help her tackle her anxiety, (i) a programme of graded exposure, (ii) challenging her appraisal that other people are staring at her and (iii) challenging her catastrophic interpretations of her physiological symptoms of anxiety.

Drawing up the programme of graded exposure involved starting with what she could cope with and emphasising that the steps involved would be small. This was as much to allay her mother's fears as it was for Jean. Ordinarily, Jean relied on her mother's support to get out and her mother remained anxious that if Jean was put under too much pressure then she would become distressed. To make the idea of a programme of graded exposure more tangible, a ladder was drawn, starting with places at the bottom where she felt 'safest' and gradually moving to places she found 'harder' to be. Time was spent discussing the order and what steps were most manageable. For instance, one step was going into a café and sitting in a quiet corner and the next step was to sit in a busier part of the café. Great care was taken to ensure that all the practical arrangements were agreed in advance for each of the outings. This included writing down when, where and who Jean would go with.

Jean was asked to record, with the help of her mother, how anxious she felt before she went out, how anxious she felt when she was out and how she felt when she got home. A simple five-point visual scale was used, of the kind described in Chap. 4, with blocks of increasing size.

Recording her feelings allowed her to reflect on how her ratings changed as she became more relaxed when she was going out and the change in her ratings as the sessions progressed.

Jean brought diary sheets with her to sessions, which her mother had helped her to complete. Through the use of thought bubbles and role play, the therapist worked with Jean on her catastrophic evaluation of her somatic symptoms of anxiety. This involved looking at the 'worst thing' that could happen and the helpful and unhelpful aspects of being a cautious person.

The other element of work addressed her fear that other people were staring at her and her belief that they probably thought she 'shouldn't be there'. In turn, this made her think that she needed 'to stop looking at people and leave as quickly as possible before she had a complete panic and made a fool of herself'. The aim was to help her become aware that her safety behaviour of looking down actually made her more anxious, because then she didn't know what was actually happening and was just left with her 'upsetting thoughts and the feelings of panic in her body'. The effect of this catastrophic thinking was drawn out, with the anxious thoughts becoming bigger and BIGGER and BIGGER.

The next session introduced a series of role plays about dropping her safety behaviour of avoiding eye contact. An accompanying homework task asked her to report what she observed was happening around her when she went out. Due to her limited literacy skills, she was asked to record her observations on a simple dictaphone that she was taught to use.

The final piece of work concerned her general confidence and her concern that other people would stare at her. She had a particular fear of travelling on buses when school children were around. She had been called names by school children in the past and was fearful that it would happen again. This was not an unrealistic fear so one component of the therapeutic work concerned boosting her self-confidence and this included reflecting on her strengths and how she thought she was viewed by others who knew her. Helpful thoughts that were elicited were rehearsed, so that she could bring them to mind when she was out (e.g. 'I have people on my side', 'Lots of people like me'). This work ended by considering the practical steps she could take to deal with people who ill-treated her. The aim was to allow her to feel confident enough to begin using buses again, initially supported by her mother.

A major motivation for Jean was her wish to meet and socialise with other people of her own age group. She wanted to get out and 'enjoy herself' again. So the therapist made contact with a worker in her community team who tried to find work or other purposeful daytime activity for clients. A link was also made with a local voluntary organisation that offers social opportunities for people with intellectual disabilities.

Tips

- When carrying out graded exposure with clients we are asking them to put themselves in anxiety-provoking situations. This makes it especially important to ensure they are motivated to embark on this work and that they understand the rationale for what they are being asked to do.
- It is usually best to start by observing your client in vivo, to gain insight into how they cope in anxiety-provoking situations.
- It is often helpful to work alongside other colleagues (e.g. nurses or occupational therapists) who provide outreach support to clients, as they can monitor the use of graded exposure strategies and ensure that the pace is appropriate.
- It might be helpful to see clients more frequently to maintain the momentum of graded exposure work.

Dealing with Setbacks

Life carries on for clients in the course of a CBT intervention. What is interesting about most books concerning CBT is that they are focused, quite understandably, on what happens in therapy. Indeed, a great deal of the language used would suggest that the clients' wider life experiences and circumstances have limited bearing on the course of the therapeutic intervention. Terms like 'dose effectiveness' make it appear as if attending therapy sessions is similar to taking medication. Of course, in reality, a range and combination of factors will lead to an individual's mental health improving or deteriorating while they are engaged in CBT. Relationship difficulties, illness or having money problems can all set someone back, while a new friendship, finding work or having a holiday or special occasion to look forward to can all improve someone's mood.

When there are setbacks it can be quite demotivating for the therapist, who can feel that their work has been ineffectual. One of the goals of CBT therapy is to try and help someone avoid becoming trapped in a cycle of despair or conflict, should difficulties arise. It may be that the client just needs a reminder of successful strategies or a recap of earlier work, to allow them to resolve their difficulties. However, if it becomes apparent that the current formulation and therapeutic plan are not working, then it may well be necessary to adjust the individual's formulation, in line with an evolving understanding of their difficulties. Once again, though, it would be a mistake to give the impression of 'starting again', particularly when the client has already done some good work. Rather, the emphasis should be about moving on to deal with other problems that have arisen. Having clear records of positive change can also be very helpful at these times and ensure that progress made is neither forgotten about nor downplayed.

Jean's Progress
Jean had been making excellent progress. She was going out most days and had joined an arts group that she attended once a week. Her overall score on the Glasgow Depression Scale had reduced to 11/30, below the clinical threshold. There were still times she felt anxious about going out but we agreed that she

was unlikely to become someone who didn't have worries and certainly not someone who wouldn't a have a care in the world. It was emphasised that low levels of anxiety are a normal part of ordinary life for many people. The main thing was that she felt more confident, was coping with getting out on a regular basis and was proud of her achievements. She even reached the stage where her mother was taking her into the town and leaving her to meet her friend for a coffee and then coming back to get her. Unfortunately, there was a major setback when she had arranged to visit a new café with her friend. It turned out the café was on the top floor of a city centre shop with picture windows overlooking hills at the edge of the city. Jean has a fear of heights and began to panic. The situation was made worse when a group of boisterous young people came into the cafe and she thought they were staring at her friend, who has Down syndrome. Jean left before she managed to finish her coffee. Whilst it initially appeared that Jean had coped with this setback well, the therapist received a call several weeks later to tell her that Jean was too anxious to leave her house and attend the therapy session. Jean's mother was concerned that it may be too much for Jean to continue with therapy when she was feeling so anxious. So the therapist agreed to go to Jean's house and they spent time recapping on the work they had done and reviewed the progress that had been made. Jean and her mum seemed to find this helpful but it was agreed to repeat some of the earlier steps, to help her leave the house again.

Finishing Therapy

Finishing therapy can be a particular challenge when the client has few confiding relationships and has built up a strong rapport with the therapist. Therapy sessions might have become a significant part of the client's week, particularly when someone has little happening in their life and few close relationships, let alone confiding relationships. As stated previously, we know from our own research (Pert et al. 2012) that some clients are looking for long-term supportive relationships rather than a time-limited intervention. So it's very important to be clear from the outset that therapy is time-limited. Unlike general adult mental health services, where the number of appointments for different manualised interventions are set for all clients, the number of sessions for clients with intellectual disabilities should be adjusted in line with what's achievable for each person. Clearly, this still has to remain within reasonable limits but a typical range would be between 10 and 20 sessions. The time-limited nature of therapy should be underlined by agreeing on the number of sessions you are going to have and by counting down when you are reaching the end of therapy. Having concrete behavioural goals that you are working towards can also help to identify a clear end point. Sometimes it can be a good idea to have a staggered finish, gradually increasing the time between sessions. This allows the client to have confidence that they have achieved change and are managing, and allows the therapist to respond to any setbacks and help the client to generalise the new skills learned.

Of course, there may be times when the client has had enough and wants to finish early or therapy stops early for other reasons. In truth, it is highly unlikely that all clients' difficulties will be overcome from a time-limited therapy like CBT, particularly as they have limited agency to control the direction of their lives. For this reason, an updated booklet can be given to clients at the close of therapy, outlining the approaches that have proved successful and with suggestions for maintaining or building on the progress that has been made. An example of the final booklet produced for Jean can be found on the website www.toolsfortalking.wordpress.com.

Working with Different Presentations and Challenges

Clearly, some of the principles and techniques that we have described in this chapter can be applied to different presentations and difficulties. What is sometimes called a *transdiagnostic* approach can offer a helpful framework for addressing a range of emotional problems and overcomes the difficulty of trying to diagnose a particular emotional problem when, in fact, people rarely have a specific disorder.

Setting out with a preconceived idea about the nature of people's difficulties can also result in the therapist making assumptions about the approach that is required and failing to consider what matters to the client. For example, in the trial of group anger management by Paul Willner et al. (2013), it was found that almost a third of their sample were clinically depressed and two-thirds had clinically significant anxiety problems. This begs the question as to whether addressing the depression, rather than the anger of those with low mood, would have been equally or more helpful for those concerned?

Yet it is undeniably the case that different problems require a slightly different approach. As already stated in Chap. 2, most research in this field concerns anger management and people with learning disabilities. There is an important book by John Taylor and Ray Novaco (2005) detailing an anger management approach based on Cognitive Behavioural Principles. John Rose and Paul Willner have also led a series of influential studies concerning group-based anger management work based on an excellent manual that sets out a series of engaging and helpful tasks for people with intellectual disabilities (Willner et al. 2013). So it is worth taking time to consider how the approach might subtly differ when addressing different difficulties.

Key Points
- Being creative can be the key to the success of a CBT intervention and is about helping clients imagine different ways of thinking and behaving.
- Behavioural change can be more tangible for clients but it needs to be part of the wider formulation that links behaviour to clients' perceptions of self and the world.
- Emotions fuel actions, so just thinking differently is not enough.
- Stigma and identity—don't ignore clients' social circumstances. Working to build more positive social identities can also be about helping them to make changes in the real world too.
- Be realistic about what can be achieved in therapy and remember that it is possible to leave clients and their supporters with a roadmap for continuing change.

References

Baron-Cohen, S. (1992). Out of sight or out of mind? Another look at deception in autism. *Journal of Child Psychology and Psychiatry, 33,* 1141–1155.

Edgerton, R. B. (1967). *The cloak of competence*. Berkeley: University of California Press.

Haslam, S. A. (2014). Making good theory practical: Five lessons for an applied social identity approach to challenges of organizational, health, and clinical psychology. *British Journal of Social Psychology, 53*(1), 1–20.

Jahoda, A., & Markova, I. (2004). Coping with social stigma: People with intellectual disabilities moving from institutions and the family home. *Journal of Intellectual Disability Research, 48*(8), 719–729.

Jahoda, A., Trower, P., Pert, C., & Fin, D. (2001). Contingent reinforcement or defending the self? A review of evolving models of aggression in people with mild learning disabilities. *British Journal of Medical Psychology, 74*, 305–321.

Jahoda, A., Selkirk, M., Trower, P., Pert, C., Stenfert Kroese, B., Dagnan, D., & Burford, B. (2009). The balance of power in therapeutic interactions with individuals who have intellectual disabilities. *British Journal of Clinical Psychology, 48*(1), 63–77. ISSN 0144-6657.

Jahoda, A., Wilson, A., Stalker, K., & Cairney, A. (2010). Living with stigma and the self-perceptions of people with mild intellectual disabilities. *Journal of Social Issues, 66*(3), 521–534. ISSN 0022-4537.

Kandel, E. (2012). *The age of insight: The quest to understand the unconscious in art, mind, and brain from Vienna 1900 to the present*. New York: Random House.

Lindsay, W. R., Jahoda, A., & Willner, P. (2013). Adapting psychological therapies for people with intellectual disabilities II. In J. T. Taylor, W. R. Lindsay, C. Hatton, & R. Hastings (Eds.), *Psychological therapies for adults with intellectual disabilities*. Oxford: Wiley/Blackwell.

Lindsay, W. R., Tinsley, S., Beail, N., Hastings, R. P., Jahoda, A., Taylor, J. L., & Hatton, C. (2015). A preliminary controlled trial of a trans-diagnostic programme for cognitive behaviour therapy with adults with intellectual disability. *Journal of Intellectual Disability Research, 59*, 360–369. doi:10.1111/jir.12145.

Linell, P., Gustavsson, L., & Juvonen, P. (1988). Interactional dominance in dyadic communication: A presentation of initiative-response analysis. *Linguistics, 26*(3), 415–442.

Pert, C., Jahoda, A., Stenfert Kroese, B., Trower, P., Dagnan, D., & Selkirk, M. (2012). Cognitive behavioural therapy from the perspective of clients with mild intellectual disabilities: A qualitative investigation of process issues. *Journal of Intellectual Disability Research, 57*, 359–369. doi:10.1111/j.1365-2788.2012.01546.x.

Spain, D., Sin, J., Chalder, T., et al. (2014). Cognitive behavior therapy for adults with autism spectrum disorders and psychiatric co-morbidity: A review. *Research in Autism Spectrum Disorders, 9*, 151–162.

Taylor, J. L., & Novaco, R. W. (2005). *Anger treatment for people with developmental disabilities: A theory, evidence and manual based approach.* New York: Wiley.

Willner, P., Rose, J., Jahoda, A., Stenfert Kroese, B., Felce, D., Cohen, D., MacMahon, P., Stimpson, A., Rose, N., Gillespie, D., Shead, J., Lammie, C., Woodgate, C., Townson, J., Nuttall, J., & Hood, K. (2013). Outcomes of a cluster-randomized controlled trial of a group-based cognitive behavioural anger management intervention for people with mild to moderate intellectual disabilities. *British Journal of Psychiatry, 203*, 288–296.

7

And Another Thing… Adapting Therapy for Particular Cognitive Impairments

Throughout this book we have discussed how CBT may need to be modified because of clients' poor attention, memory problems, communication or rigid thinking. The nature and extent of impairments will differ from one client to another, and will not necessarily be obvious at the outset of therapy. So the therapist has to be flexible, creative and willing to navigate some unexpected twists and turns as therapy proceeds.

We thought it would be worthwhile pausing to reflect further on some of the most common cognitive impairments and consider some adjustments the therapist might make, although we don't want to suggest that the hurdles faced in therapy are all due to clients' intellectual disabilities. A client who strays off topic during sessions may be displaying problems of attention and distractibility, or may be avoiding conversations that he or she finds uncomfortable or upsetting. So the therapist must keep an open mind about the root cause of these difficulties before deciding on the best way forward.

We start by giving a broad outline of difficulties encountered when working with problems of poor memory, attention and communication and consider some adjustments the therapist might make. We end the chapter with a case study, showing how therapy with one client was obstructed by the client's rigid thinking style.

© The Author(s) 2017
B. Stenfert Kroese et al., *Cognitive Behaviour Therapy for People with Intellectual Disabilities*, DOI 10.1057/978-1-137-47854-2_7

Working with Memory Problems

As mentioned in Chap. 4, the majority of clients with intellectual disabilities will be unable to recall detailed historical information, so the therapist often has to gather background information from carers or family members. An additional challenge when working with clients who have specific memory difficulties is that they may be unable to recall recent experiences, impacting on the quality of information brought to therapy sessions. Memory problems can also affect the carry-over of information from one session to another, slowing down the pace of therapy and limiting the scope of what can be achieved in each session. An added problem is that clients can feel embarrassed or discouraged by their inability to recall information, which can ultimately impact on self-efficacy and engagement. Some clients may attempt to cover up their difficulties by using guesswork or becoming acquiescent. Memory issues can also lead to poor attendance at appointments due to forgetfulness, or failure to complete self-monitoring tasks for the same reason. Some techniques to work with memory issues are presented below.

> **Box 7.1 Adaptations to CBT When Working with Memory Problems**
>
> - Gather background information from a carer who knows the client well. Draw up a visual timeline of events chunked into categories that make sense to your client (e.g. when I was a child/when I was at school/when I was at college/when I moved into my own flat). This can be used as a focus point during sessions.
> - Ask carers to support the client with homework and diaries.
> - Deliver the information in small chunks to keep the demands on your client's memory to a minimum. Use short, catchy slogans (e.g. 'think calm – feel calm') for easier recall.
> - Back up verbal information with visual illustration as your client may retain this more easily. Draw up visual cue cards that clients can carry with them as a memory prompt. Ensure that these are portable and accessible. A popular option is putting cue cards on a key ring.
> - Develop colourful, eye-catching materials that are individualised for each client (e.g. using pictures of the clients' favourite television character or pet), as these will be more memorable.
> - Recap on key information repeatedly throughout each session.

- Introduce memory prompts (e.g. a sticker on the fridge) and other cues to remind your client to fill out their diary.
- Give your client a 'therapy pack' to collate all information in order to aid recall.
- Normalise memory problems to avoid your client becoming discouraged.

Problems of Attention and Distractibility

Clients with poor attention are likely to struggle to remain focused throughout a standard hour-long therapy session, causing them to either 'zone out' or become distracted. A common difficulty is that clients stray off the topic of conversation on to other subjects, disrupting the flow of sessions. This can be particularly difficult when conducting appointments in the client's own home where the therapist has no control over distractions. When it is necessary to repeatedly redirect a client back on to topic there can be a risk of the client feeling reprimanded or criticised, which can impact negatively on the therapeutic relationship. One way of managing these interruptions is by using the session agenda to redirect the conversation back onto the session plan, or to set aside time at the end of sessions for clients' own 'off topic' discussion. We find that asking clients to delay a conversation until later is more comfortable than asking them to 'shut down' the topic altogether. Other adaptations overlap with those used for memory problems such as slowing down the pace of sessions and delivering information in small manageable chunks. These and other suggestions are summarised below.

Box 7.2 Adaptations to CBT for Poor Attention and Distractibility
- Keep sessions shorter and pace information according to the client's needs.
- Use visual aids to 'grab' attention and offer a break from verbal dialogue, for example, individualised photographs or 'Tools for Talking' (Unwin et al. 2016).
- Use the CBT session agenda as a reference point to return a distractible client back on to the session topic.

> - Introduce ways for your client to be actively involved, such as by ticking off agenda items as the session proceeds.
> - Establish frequent 'check in' points during sessions to make sure you are progressing through the agenda items.
> - If your client strays off on to different topics, set aside time at the end of the session and redirect 'off topic' discussion to that slot.
> - Ensure that therapy sessions are held in a setting that is free from distractions.

Communication Difficulties

Common communication difficulties include both verbal comprehension and expressive problems, such as articulation difficulties and limited vocabulary. When there is a disparity between a client's expressive skills and their comprehension, there is a risk that the therapist might over- or underestimate their ability.

It can interrupt the momentum of therapy sessions and jeopardise rapport and engagement when the therapist repeatedly fails to understand what their client has said, although, in our experience, the majority of clients prove to be patient and persistent in their efforts to be understood. This will be boosted by a therapist who remains relaxed, respectful and encouraging. If you can't understand your client's speech, it may help to ask questions that range from the very general, using your best guesses and only requiring the client to nod or point. Or you might ask the client to choose options from cue cards or a multiple choice task on a flip chart. For instance, you might break the options down into a series of two choices such as 'is this about something that happened at 1/home or 2/at work?' and then 'was it something 1/your mother did or was it 2/someone else?'

Some clues to look out for are when the client repeatedly answers 'yes' to all questions, which could indicate that they don't understand the question, are unable to find an answer or wish to please the therapist by agreeing.

Clients may display other idiosyncratic social communication problems such as poor turn taking skills, poor interpersonal boundaries or an inability to read non-verbal cues. Interpersonal styles can vary greatly, from the client who talks in a one-sided fashion and has poor listening skills, to those who may be quietly spoken, reticent and need encouragement to join in. In both cases the challenge for the therapist is to achieve a balanced clinical conversation. This could mean tightening the structure of sessions to contain a talkative client, or taking time to slowly build trust with a client who is unresponsive. A range of ways the therapist might support communication difficulties are listed below.

> **Box 7.3 Adaptations to CBT When Working with Communication Problems**
> - Use simple language and words that are familiar to the client. Use the client's own preferred terminology where possible. Use concrete language and avoid abstract concepts.
> - If you have difficulty understanding what your client has said you can ask a series of questions to narrow down the options. The client can confirm or reject these options. Alternatively, use a multiple choice task on a flip chart.
> - If your client has sufficient communication ability use open-ended questions to overcome acquiescence and encourage full responses.
> - Give real-life examples to aid understanding where possible.
> - Present information in different formats. Use visual materials to support understanding and make use of gestures (e.g. thumbs up), facial expression and active methods. Real objects can also be used to aid communication.
> - To override the need for clients to respond verbally, sort cue cards into categories, or write multiple choice options on a flip chart. Resources such as photo symbols or 'Tools for Talking' (Unwin et al. 2016) can also be used flexibly.
> - Invite a family member or carer who knows the client well to join sessions, or parts of sessions, to support communication problems.
> - Establish a plan at the outset to deal with communication difficulties, such as agreeing that you can both ask each other to repeat what was said.
> - For turn taking difficulties agree on a cue to indicate when the therapist wishes to talk.
> - You might ask your client (in a relaxed, non-threatening way) to summarise what has been said to check their understanding.

Problems of Cognitive Rigidity

The key CBT objective of reconstructing clients' appraisals is compromised when working with clients who have a rigid cognitive style. Even when motivated to work on their emotional difficulties, clients with this cognitive style often remain stuck on their current views and resistant to the therapists' suggestions that they should adjust their thinking. The following case study describes therapy with Alan, who has anger problems and a rigid thinking style.

Presenting Problem

Alan is aged 32 years and has a mild intellectual disability. His anger problems are long-standing, but exacerbated recently due to his conflict with a neighbour when she came to his door to complain about noise from his television. Alan became verbally aggressive, which resulted in his neighbour making a complaint to the housing department. This incident happened some months prior to the referral; however, Alan continued to ruminate and engage in cyclical discussions about the incident. He had become convinced that he and his mother would be evicted from their home.

Clinical Interview and Background Information

Alan is an only child who has lived at home with his mother throughout his life. Alan previously had a close relationship with his grandfather who died three years ago.

During early clinical sessions Alan was invited by the therapist to talk about his life experiences, telling his own story. He spoke of being badly bullied at school and being picked on by people in the local neighbourhood. His grandfather encouraged him to fight back, and criticised him for not doing so, telling him he was weak (rules for living: to tolerate injustice is weak). Alan attended college after leaving school but got into arguments with other students and was excluded due to being aggressive in class. This fuelled a sense of injustice as Alan saw his aggression as justified, as it was in response to taunting from other students.

Alan described himself as a good person, saying he is a good son and was a loyal grandson. He spoke of a sense of self-worth which he felt when helping his grandfather with tasks such as food shopping and housework. He has a close relationship with his mother and benefits from her support with his current problem. Again, he spoke proudly of the fact that he helps his mother at home.

Alan has led an isolated life with no lasting friendships. He would like to have friends but he is also wary about meeting new people and is suspicious of people's motives. He has very few opportunities to socialise with peers as he doesn't have any regular planned activities. He rarely goes out without his mother, although he is able to travel independently.

Alan's mother also has a very limited support network since the death of her father who she had previously depended on for practical and emotional support. She has found it difficult to deal with Alan's fixation with their neighbour and tends to respond by reassuring Alan that the argument wasn't his fault.

Self-Monitoring

Alan was asked to keep a diary every time he felt angry, rating the severity on a three-point scale and stating the trigger to his anger (see the website www.toolsfortalking.wordpress.com). Alan's diary entries confirmed that his anger was most often linked with rumination over the recent complaint from his neighbour. The diaries also showed that Alan was in the habit of questioning his mother about the likely outcome of their neighbour's complaint to the housing officer, which often led to increased anger.

Social Understanding

As described in Chap. 4, storyboards were used to identify Alan's social cognitive skills and to explore themes in Alan's appraisals of interpersonal situations (Pert and Jahoda 2008; Jahoda et al. 2006). Stories about a range of relevant topics including being treated unfairly (*having your drink stolen*) or incidents of accidental harm (*someone accidentally spilling a drink over you*) allowed exploration of Alan's understanding of the emotions and actions of the characters in the story. It was also possible to explore more sophisticated skills such as Alan's understanding of the characters' intentions (*Was it an accident or deliberate?*) and his ability to take on the different points of view of the various characters in the stories. Themes that arose in his understanding of what occurred were also noted, to identify possible biases in his thinking, such as a tendency to assume hostility, or misinterpret others' actions. The storyboard approach was also useful to explore Alan's view of different ways of dealing with social difficulties, such as aggression, assertiveness and submissiveness. The focus on other characters in the stories rather than himself was helpful as a starting point as Alan spoke more openly and was less defensive. The findings of this exercise are shown below.

- Alan was able to identify the characters' emotions and behaviour with no difficulty.
- Alan presented an 'all or nothing' global thinking style when interpreting the stories tending to view the characters as globally good or bad.
- He was unable to shift his perspective in light of new information offered.
- Alan was shown to have limited perspective-taking ability, which might explain his difficulty appreciating the viewpoint of his neighbour.
- Alan viewed aggressive behaviour as a way of showing strength and an acceptable strategy when dealing with provocation. This was also partly due to his dichotomous thinking, believing it was fair to hurt others who had hurt him.

Identifying Helpful and Unhelpful Thoughts

The link between Alan's thoughts and feelings was explored in clinical discussions where a flip chart was used to draw out a thinking, feeling and behaviour cycle. As it was difficult to elicit Alan's thoughts in this way, the therapist also used role play to act out the argument with Alan's neighbour, stopping him mid role play to explore what was going through his mind at the time. The therapist guided Alan to practice alternative calm thoughts and 'act out' how calm thinking would make him feel and what he would then do. Alan was gradually encouraged to identify his own calm thoughts.

The following appraisal and beliefs were identified:

> **CBT Appraisals and Beliefs**
>
> *Appraisal:* 'She doesn't like me and is trying to get me evicted.'
> *Evaluative beliefs:* 'She is unjust and against me in every way.'
> *Core Beliefs:* 'I am a victim.'
> 'Others are hostile and not trustworthy.'
> 'I must fight back otherwise I'm weak.'
> *Behavioural Consequences:* Alan defends himself by 'fighting back' to get justice, which can involve shouting and swearing at others, and sometimes throwing objects.
> *Thinking Style:* Alan presents a global thinking style, 'right versus wrong/good versus bad' and a tendency to get stuck on fixed ideas and ruminate.

Aspects of Alan's Presentation that Obstructed Therapy

There were a number of barriers to progress identified during assessment, including Alan's ambivalence about the need for change. As Alan viewed himself as being a victim, he found it difficult to accept the need for change ('It was her fault not mine'). This was partly addressed by sharing an accessible formulation with Alan that highlighted the benefits of change (see later in this chapter). Given his ambivalence it was particularly important that the therapeutic goals set were meaningful and acceptable to Alan. Goals agreed by Alan were to work on 'reducing worry' and 'show that I'm strong'.

Aspects of Alan's thinking style, including his cognitive rigidity and tendency to get stuck in a loop of cyclical discussions during sessions, obstructed both the process and the content of sessions. Where possible, the therapist accommodated Alan's rigid thinking style by using concrete language and bipolar constructs (was it helpful or unhelpful; were you calm or angry?). However, his rigid thinking style meant that Alan continued to find it difficult to reframe and reconstruct his appraisals. A typical example of Alan's dichotomous reasoning was that he viewed each appraisal as either 'truth or lies'. This meant that accepting alternative appraisals to his own would mean he was 'a liar'. Being a liar would mean he was a bad person, which ran counter to his self-identity (I'm a good, loyal, strong person).

Alan's inability to accept alternative appraisals led to him becoming defensive during sessions when asked to consider a different way of looking at things. Again, he saw this as evidence that the therapist thought he was 'a liar', which led to minor disengagement during some sessions. To overcome Alan's defensiveness and maintain rapport, the therapist emphasised the collaborative approach, working together 'as a team' to achieve the therapeutic goals set out earlier.

Alan's defensiveness was also linked with his self-identity, particularly his need to be viewed by others as a good person. This in turn contributed to his sensitivity to being blamed and resistance to accept alternative appraisals. This could be picked up later by the therapist when working on calm thinking, by focusing on self-affirming thoughts, such as being a good person and a strong resilient person, that matched Alan's self-perceptions.

After four sessions a draft formulation shown below was drawn up using the 5 *P*'s model, already discussed in Chap. 5.

Draft Formulation

Presenting problem
Alan was referred with problems of anger and anxiety, characterised by problems of rumination.

Precipitating factors
Alan became 'stuck' on concerns of injustice following a neighbour's complaint regarding noise.

Predisposing factors
Early experiences of bullying and ridicule from others, had led to Alan seeing the world as unfair, and others as hostile and unfriendly. Alan was encouraged to use aggressive strategies by his grandfather when he was a child, and he learned that aggression was a way of gaining respect. Due to Alan's concrete, rigid thinking style he views events in a polarised fashion and is unable to reappraise events. This leads to him becoming stuck on his views and resistant to alternative appraisals.

Perpetuating factors
Alan's anger and aggressiveness is driven by a sense of injustice, and desire to gain respect by a show of strength. However, aggressive strategies have led to problems with housing and previous exclusion from college, which have further reinforced his sense of injustice and powerlessness. Alan's tendency to ruminate over situations of conflict and get stuck in repetitive thought loops also fuels his anger. A lack of friendships and social opportunities further fosters a sense of alienation and injustice.

Protective factors
Alan's desire to be a good person and his wish to develop positive peer relationships and increase his social opportunities offer a basis on which to build towards change. His close relationship with his mother offers stability and support.

Feeding Back an Accessible Formulation

To enhance Alan's understanding of his problems and provide a rationale for change, a more accessible version of the formulation was developed and shared with Alan. To ensure it was easy to understand, some of the contributing factors contained in the full formulation were not included in this accessible version (such as cognitive style, core beliefs and self-perceptions).

> **Accessible Formulation**
>
> *You have always lived with your mum and you both spend a lot of time together at home. You would like friends but it hasn't been easy to meet a good friend.*
>
> *You've been treated badly by people in the past and that made you feel hurt. That means than you learned to look out for bad treatment and stick up for yourself.*
>
> *BUT the way you stick up for yourself can lead to more problems, because sometimes you end up in trouble and fall out with people. Falling out with people can leave you feeling lonely at times. Then you feel even worse—so you find that getting mad with people doesn't always help you.*
>
> *You have a lot of time at home with nothing to do, so you spend a lot of time worrying about things that have happened, and sometimes worries get stuck in your head, such as 'she is against me' and 'I've been treated badly'.*
>
> *Thinking these thoughts makes you feel **even more** worried and **even more** angry.*
>
> *So your problems just get worse and worse.*

The therapist presented this formulation as a working document, emphasising that Alan could make changes, or give his own ideas. The formulation was chunked into sections to aid understanding and help Alan discriminate between causal factors relating to his past experience and those relating to his aggression, rumination and angry thoughts. The formulation was written on a flipchart with arrows showing the links between contributing factors and Alan's anger. Overall, Alan responded well to the draft formulation. The link made between his early experiences of bullying and his current anger and aggression made sense to him. This appeared to reassure him that his anger problem wasn't seen as his 'fault' and he wasn't being judged or blamed, which was consistent with his view of himself as a good person.

As is often the case, the process of feeding back the formulation led to improved rapport and engagement, as Alan had a clear rationale for moving forward. Alan's mother was invited to join the formulation feedback session in order to share the formulation with her and agree on a plan to support Alan when he was ruminating or engaging in repetitive questioning about his neighbour.

The accessible formulation offered a way of highlighting to Alan that his current ways of coping made things worse for himself, and therefore he should try out new techniques. It was agreed that Alan's ongoing anger and worry was causing him to lose out in life which wasn't fair on him, and that he deserved a break from these worries. Aggression was reframed as *losing control* and staying calm was reframed as *staying in control* to overcome Alan's view that aggression is effective and strong. Externalising strategies were used, agreeing that he 'shouldn't let anger beat him'. To improve motivation further, Alan and the therapist made a list of benefits that would result from staying calm, including having less worry in life, feeling proud and staying out of trouble with the housing department.

Intervention. A Concrete Plan

Following the above rationale for change, it was agreed that Alan would use a new coping plan, which he called 'a fresh start'.

Making the Thinking Feeling Link: One Thing Leads to Another

The CBT link between thoughts, emotions and behaviour was presented to Alan as 'one thing leads to another' and presented in pictorial form as seen in the Fresh Start booklet (see www.toolsfortalking.wordpress.com). To aid recall a slogan 'Think Calm, Feel Calm' was agreed and rehearsed frequently during sessions.

However, due to Alan's rigid thinking, he continued to get 'stuck' on his views and had difficulty letting go of his angry thinking. As mentioned earlier, he saw his thoughts as being 'the truth' and found it difficult to understand that his own thoughts may be fuelling his anger. Given this, when exploring the negative impact of Alan's thinking, rather than focusing directly on the dispute with his neighbour the therapist began by using a neutral story (see storyboards earlier). What would Alan think about events depicting someone else in a similar situation? Ultimately the aim of this was to demonstrate to Alan that there was more than one way of looking at things.

Guidance Towards Reappraisal

Rather than identifying alternative appraisals in the usual way, a more guided approach was needed. Options were suggested by the therapist based on themes that had arisen during role play, clinical discussions and the storyboard exercise. It had been established that Alan viewed his neighbour as being 'against me' and 'a bully', so the therapist reframed this to suggest a contrasting view that his neighbour may have been stressed or scared when Alan shouted at her, which then led to her complaining to the housing officer. It was hoped that this reappraisal would reduce Alan's view that his neighbour was bullying him and therefore reduce his sense of threat and fears about future harassment. The therapist also attempted to redress Alan's catastrophic view (*we will definitely be evicted*), by disputing that this was a definite outcome as opposed to something that was possible, but unlikely. To further reduce his sense of inevitability about eviction, Alan was asked to think about ways that he could improve relationships with his housing officer and his neighbour to resolve the situation. However, despite some progress, it was difficult to sustain alternative views and Alan continued to fall back on catastrophic thinking.

How True on a Scale of 0–10?

The therapist attempted to reduce the *strength* of Alan's belief that his neighbour was against him, by focusing on positive interactions he had with his neighbour in the past. Alan was able to recall a number of positive exchanges, such as when given a Christmas card and an offer of help with heavy bags. There was some limited shift in Alan's belief which he now rated as 8/10 true as opposed to a previous rating of 10/10.

Given Alan's resistance, the therapist decided to focus mainly on the rehearsal of calm thinking rather than challenging Alan's current appraisals further. Further input regarding the negative impact of angry thinking could then be introduced later in therapy if there was scope to do so.

As Alan was unable to generate his own calm thoughts, a number of options were suggested to him, based on themes that had emerged from clinical discussion, storyboards and role play. Alan choose from a selection of self-affirming thoughts ('I'm a good person; I can stay proud') and thoughts about resilience and being in control ('I've got through difficult times before', 'I can stay strong and steady; I won't let anger beat me').

Balanced Thinking

To demonstrate Alan's tendency to ruminate on unhelpful thoughts, the therapist used a set of balanced weighing scales and explained to Alan that one side of the scales represented angry thinking and the other side calm thinking. Coloured cue cards (heavy weighted cards) were used and angry thoughts (red) or calm thoughts (blue) were written on each. Alan was asked to identify which side each card belonged. Alan's angry thoughts were placed on one side of the scales causing the scales to become off balance. Alternate calm thoughts were written on blue cards and placed on the other side of the scale to demonstrate that calm thoughts had an opposite effect (see below).

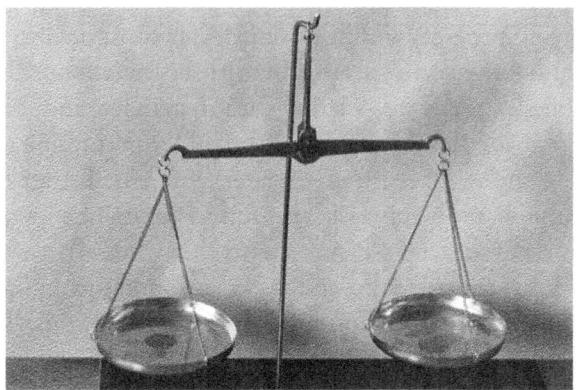

This concrete, active technique corresponded well with Alan's tendency to see things in a polarised way (angry or calm) and helped him to see how one-sided and out of balance his thinking was. By using a tangible, interactive technique Alan was able to understand how angry thinking could be brought back into balance by thinking calm thoughts. So rather than asking Alan to cease angry thoughts, which he was resistant to do, the strategy was to actively rehearse calm thoughts.

But How Does This Work in Real Life?

Given Alan's rigid thinking, he was likely to have difficulty generalising strategies from the therapy room to real life; and from one real-life situation to another. So, the next step was to use role play to demonstrate how the calm thoughts that had been identified would help in day-to-day stressful situations, such as Alan meeting his neighbour in the local streets or shops. This allowed Alan to choose the best calm thoughts for each situation. The role plays increased his understanding of the thinking feeling link and left him feeling more confident and prepared to deal with these situations when they arose. When the benefits of calm thinking had been established using role play, the therapist introduced the rehearsal of assertive coping strategies during role play to offer alternatives to aggression keeping in mind Alan's belief that if he didn't stand up for himself he was weak.

Getting Stuck on Thoughts

Despite showing progress within sessions Alan continued to spend time at home ruminating on the argument with his neighbour. Rumination was undoubtedly partly associated with inactivity and boredom, so attempts were made to introduce more purpose and routine to Alan's life by a referral to the social services (see later). An added strategy of 'taking a break from your problems' was also introduced and supported by his mother at times of difficulty. It was agreed that when Alan was unable to break out of his ruminative thought cycle his mother would prompt him to use a distraction activity, choosing from a list of options. These strategies were summarised and illustrated in booklet form and can be found on the website www.toolsfortalking.wordpress.com.

Gaps in Therapy

Due to Alan's poor perspective-taking ability, it proved difficult for him to recognise the negative impact of his aggression on others. However, as Alan had shown a heightened sensitivity to blame, the therapist decided not to pursue this issue of empathy and perspective taking further, as there was a possibility Alan would disengage from therapy.

Progress Made

Alan's diaries suggested fewer outbursts of anger and a reduced severity of anger ratings, suggesting that Alan was able to benefit from using the balanced thinking techniques. Clinical discussions with Alan and his mother also suggested a positive impact on Alan's self-worth and sense of efficacy. He continued to ruminate and feel a sense of injustice at times, but felt more equipped to deal with this.

Real Changes Too

Alan's mother had been clearly struggling to cope in her role of carer for many years and had opted not to join weekly therapy sessions, perhaps due to her own difficulties. It was clear that her limited support network and lack of opportunity to be more active outwith the home was a significant contributing factor. With their consent, the therapist referred Alan and his mother to social work services, who carried out a carer's assessment and referred Alan to a local community drop-in group where he volunteered in a community garden project with support from project workers. It was hoped that this would give Alan a valued role, and offer an opportunity to develop peer relationships in a safe context. The social worker also liaised with the housing department to work towards a resolution of the issue with Alan's neighbour.

To finish therapy the therapist pulled together the key strategies together in a booklet (see the website www.toolsfortalking.wordpress.com), which would aid Alan's recall and also offer a reference point for his mother to support him with these strategies.

A summary of the adaptations that can help to overcome cognitive rigidity are shown below.

> **Adaptations to CBT When Working with a Rigid Thinking Style**
> - Clarify whether your client's cognitive rigidity and 'stuckness' is related to a specific cognitive deficit by using an assessment of social understanding. A storyboard showing interactions between two characters can be used to explore your client's understanding of the emotional impact of events, ability to predict likely outcomes, understanding of others intentions and perspective taking.
> - Where appropriate accommodate your client's rigid thinking style, by talking in unambiguous 'concrete' language.
> - If your client is resistant to cognitive change, draw up a list of tangible benefits of change (e.g. staying out of trouble, less worry, feeling proud) and frequently review this with your client.
> - When establishing the CBT link between thinking and feeling, rather than focusing on your client's own unhelpful thinking start by using a 'neutral' story to demonstrate that different thoughts will lead to different feelings.
> - If your client is unable to generate alternative appraisals use a more guided approach by suggesting possible alternatives based on themes that have arisen.
> - When clients are resistant to change start by introducing helpful thoughts rather than disputing the content of the client's negative thinking. One option is to use a set of scales to demonstrate the distinction between helpful and unhelpful thinking, and show how thinking can be 'off balance'.
> - Clients with rigid thinking may have difficulty generalising strategies from one situation to another so use role play to demonstrate how techniques can be used in real-life stressful situations.

Conclusions

Whilst we hope that this chapter offers the therapist a helpful summary of adaptations, many of which we have already touched upon in previous chapters, we also want to stress that in real life the causal links, and solutions, are rarely so clear-cut or tidy. We have highlighted that often memory, attention and communication difficulties impact primarily on the therapy *process*, disrupting the flow of sessions, client engagement and affecting rapport. We have suggested some ways of working but recognise that often the way forward doesn't lie in 'techniques' alone, but rests on strong therapeutic relationships and core skills of warmth, genuineness and empathy (Bachelor and Horvath 1999). The ability to put your clients at ease and ensure they feel listened to and understood will help to get round many obstacles in therapy, irrespective of the root cause.

> **Key Points**
> - Common cognitive impairments such as poor memory, attention and communication can impact on progress during of CBT therapy.
> - The nature of adaptations required will depend on the extent of clients' problems.
> - It is the therapist's responsibility to adjust their approach to meet the needs of the client.
> - Some difficulties affect the process of therapy whilst others impact on the content of sessions and formulation.
> - A strong therapeutic relationship will help overcome problems relating to the process of therapy, such as problems with the engagement or rapport.
> - Some adaptations apply across the board such as using simple language and a slower pace and repetition.

References

Bachelor, A., & Horvath, A. (1999). The therapeutic relationship. In M. A. Hubble, B. L. Duncan, & S. D. Miller (Eds.), *The heart and soul of change: What works in therapy*. Washington, DC: American Psychological Association.

Jahoda, A., Pert, C., & Trower, P. (2006). Frequent aggression and attribution of hostile intent in people with mild to moderate intellectual disabilities: An empirical investigation. *American Journal of Mental Retardation, 111*(2), 90–99.

Pert, C., & Jahoda, A. (2008). Social goals and conflict strategies of individuals with mild to moderate intellectual disabilities who present problems of aggression. *Journal of Intellectual Disability Research, 52*(5), 393–403. doi:10.1111/j.1365-2788.2007.01039.

Unwin, G., Larkin, M., Rose, J., Stenfert Kroese, B., & Malcolm, S. (2016). Developing resources to facilitate culturally-sensitive service planning and delivery – Doing research inclusively with people with learning disabilities. *Research Involvement and Engagement.* doi:10.1186/s40900-016-00.

8

Group Work

We have described how to work therapeutically on a 1:1 basis, and although we have stressed the importance of involving others and the benefits of adopting systemic therapeutic techniques, the CBT approaches so far focus on one particular person with ID at a time. This chapter will introduce ways in which to use CBT principles in group work where the aim is to achieve positive psychological change for small groups of clients concurrently. We will consider the benefits as well as the barriers to successful group therapy for adults with ID.

Why Consider Group Work for People with ID?

> By the crowd they have been broken, by the crowd they shall be healed. (Marsh 1953)

When consulting the general literature on group therapy this quote often crops up. We understand that L.C. Marsh, to whom we have traced the quote, was a much-admired pioneer in the development of group therapy. He practised in this way as far back as the 1930s with therapeutic groups that consisted of people who had been labelled as 'schizophrenic'.

We think it is particularly relevant to consider Marsh's quote (and its clear reference to large numbers of perpetrators) when working with people with ID. The clients we see have often been harmed, not only by a discrete number of negative interpersonal experiences, but throughout their lives by frequent messages of being 'other' and by being on the receiving end of rejection, scorn and stigmatisation from peers and other groups they may have wanted to be part of.

So is it true, as the quote implies, that 'healing' can only be achieved by receiving therapeutic messages in a group context and that the work done by one therapist during individual therapy will have less or no impact? We believe not and consider that 1:1 CBT sessions and developing individual therapeutic relationships can have powerful beneficial effects for our clients. On the other hand, as clinicians we have also witnessed the remarkable and lasting impact of group work on some of our clients and as researchers we have been impressed with the quantitative as well as the qualitative evidence of effective therapeutic groups, and we are therefore enthusiastic advocates for this type of intervention.

There is a considerable evidence base to be found in the general mental health research literature for effective CBT group interventions for a variety of psychological problems including general anxiety, depression, bulimia, bipolar disorder, PTSD and complex trauma reactions, drug and alcohol problems, and offending behaviours including sexual offending. Delivering CBT in a group format is a cost-effective alternative to individual therapy (e.g. Vos et al. 2005), and group therapy can have further advantages, as clients benefit from group cohesion and normalisation effects and they can use the group as an arena for engaging in behavioural experiments, learning from others and functioning as co-therapists (Whitfield 2010).

Bender and Tombs (1992) talked about the benefits of the collective experience that therapy groups can provide for people with intellectual disabilities, and more than 20 years later a review of controlled trials of psychotherapeutic interventions for adults with ID (Vereenhooghe and Langdon 2013) supports his observation. The studies included in this review show that effect sizes for CBT group work can be equal to (and at times greater than) equivalent individual interventions.

One such study (Willner et al. 2013) that we have been involved in evaluated a manualised CBT group intervention for adults with intellectual disabilities who had problems with anger control. Clinical psychologists trained service staff (we called them lay therapists) across 30 different services to deliver a treatment manual and gave them fortnightly supervision throughout. Key-worker ratings on the Provocation Index (Novaco 2003) were significantly lower after the intervention, both service users and their key workers reported greater use of anger coping skills and both key workers and home carers reported lower levels of challenging behaviour after the intervention and at follow-up.

So why does group therapy work at all for people with ID? It would be reasonable to expect that when clients have to share the attention and input from their therapists with a number of others equally in need of psychological help, it would result in a 'watering down' of any therapeutic effect. We turn to the findings of researchers and the musings of commentators on the group therapies that have been on offer for the general population since the early days of Marsh to throw some light on this question.

Many therapists who report on their clinical group work talk about the influence of *non-specific* factors, in particular the role of group dynamics. They consider these dynamics to have a positive effect on how clients view their problems by normalising them and clients being made to feel supported, encouraged and not alone by their fellow group members who have also suffered and survived similar experiences. Yalom and Leszcz (2005) lists 11 ways in which groups can provide non-specific therapeutic benefits that may occur regardless of the psychological theoretical model adopted by the group therapists. They are too numerous to describe in detail but we will briefly list them in the box below because we consider that they all have an important role to play and we have observed their impact on clients with intellectual disabilities in our own clinical practice.

1. Universality (similar to normalising the problem)
2. Development of socialising techniques (gaining confidence and skills in social interaction)
3. Imparting information (factual learning from the content of the sessions)
4. Cohesiveness (positive experience of being part of a group, a feeling of belonging and mutual acceptance)
5. Interpersonal learning (listening to and learning from other group members, receiving their feedback)
6. Altruism (helping others increases self-esteem and a sense of purpose)
7. Installation of hope (being inspired and encouraged by other group members)
8. Imitative behaviours (modelling adaptive behaviours of others)
9. Existential factors (accepting that no life is free of pain and concepts of responsibility and freedom throw up complex and challenging issues)
10. Catharsis (psychological healing through talking about problems)
11. Corrective recapitulation of family experiences (understanding the impact of early experiences and learning to avoid repeating unhelpful patterns if interaction)

All these non-specific factors are said to increase motivation and active engagement within the group setting and because we consider them to be important, we feel justified in incorporating theoretical models other than CBT in our group therapy practice. We are not alone in adopting 'pragmatic blending' (Halgin 1985) and consider this to be akin to a metacompetent approach (Whittington and Grey 2014) that we have described in Chap. 2. That is, psychodynamic, interpersonal and client-centred principles can be combined with CBT principles (if they don't already overlap) in a planned rather than a haphazard way and introduced only if they are considered to be responsive to and suitable for the group members' psychological needs. For example, to uncover and explore issues that the client is not aware of you may consider techniques used by psychodynamic therapists such as asking people to free associate or to use art to represent, for example, their problems or their family.

To address problematic interpersonal styles we may consider how the relationships they develop in the group can inform and help the client to develop more adaptive ways of interacting. And we may use a client-centred approach when people struggle to share personal experiences by promoting a sense of 'caring genuineness', acceptance and empathy amongst group members.

So although the demands on our clients with intellectual disabilities are likely to be greater when we ask them to take part in group CBT rather than 1:1 CBT, we have found that for many of the people referred to us, being part of a group has additional advantages because of the non-specific factors that can help them to address personal as well as interpersonal issues.

What Do Clients Think About Groups?

While quantitative research methods can capture prescribed aspects of psychological change due to participating in an intervention, they don't always provide information about the process issues. And it often is process issues that participants perceive as more important than the specific outcomes as measured by psychometrics. McLeod (2011) argues that typical quantitative outcome studies of the effectiveness of therapy are often written up in a way 'that privileges some voices and silences others … The feelings and personal experiences of clients, therapists, supervisors and other participants in these studies are not reported at all.' He argues that qualitative research methods such as Interpretative Phenomenological Analysis (IPA Smith et al. 2009) and Thematic Analysis (Braun and Clarke 2006) that are based on social constructionist principles allow those silenced voices to be heard as they focus on identifying interpersonal processes and personal experiences. By providing opportunities for clients to have their voices heard by means of qualitative research methods, we can avoid making assumptions about their experiences of group therapy what they perceive to be the most significant and useful aspects of the intervention.

People with intellectual disabilities have relatively few opportunities to express their opinions and emotions, yet in a review as far back as 1998 'Consumers with Intellectual Disabilities as Service Evaluators' (Stenfert Kroese, Gillott and Atkinson 1998) we conclude that 'Most studies found that given adequate opportunities and effective interview methods, people with intellectual disabilities can be informative, critical and reliable service evaluators'. For this reason, the development of appropriate qualitative methodology to enable clients' voices to be sought and heard, in particular their views on and experiences of psychological interventions, is important if clinical approaches including CBT are to be advanced in an evidence-based way.

A number of authors have interviewed people with intellectual disabilities about their experiences of taking part in a CBT group. These groups were run for a variety of psychological problems including depression, anger (dealing with difficult feelings), sexual offending and complex trauma. The findings of these qualitative studies suggest that having the opportunity to talk about painful experiences and difficult problems and to be included, supported and valued in a group is much appreciated (e.g. 'Understanding that you're not on your own … It feels good'; Stenfert Kroese et al. 2016). Many people spoke about the value and joy of developing new relationships with other group members and experiencing the group as a safe place to talk and be listened to (e.g. 'I worked out that if you're swopping stories, it helps each other out'; MacMahon et al. 2015). The participants of these and other studies were able to recall many positive, helpful and at times funny exchanges. They often were particularly struck by the disclosures of the group therapists, when the therapists talked about their own problems with anger, anxiety and other psychological 'wobbles' they experienced and were prepared to share. For our client group, this appears to be a powerful way to normalise psychological distress and 'model' helpful coping strategies.

The theme 'being listened to' is widely reported when participants are asked to reflect on their experiences of individual (e.g. Pert et al. 2013) as well as group therapy (e.g. MacMahon et al. 2015). Clients often express their surprise at being taken seriously and note that the therapists appear to value their opinions and make an effort to understand their problems. The experience of being listened to and respected is compared with how in other settings they feel ignored or dismissed.

Here are some quotes taken from a paper we wrote after talking to a number of clients who attended one of three trauma-focused cognitive behavioural therapy (TF-CBT) groups (Stenfert Kroese et al. 2016). First a short description of the background information that led us to adapt this therapeutic approach is presented in the Box below.

> The psychological problems of people with intellectual disabilities who suffer PTSD are typically managed pharmacologically (although efficacy has not been demonstrated; Willner 2015) or by working behaviourally with staff teams (British Psychological Society et al. 2007). These interventions do not address the underlying causes of PTSD.
>
> CBT has been shown to be effective treatment for PTSD and a Cochrane Review (Bisson et al. 2013) concludes that individual TF-CBT is the most effective intervention for PTSD in the general adult population and that group TF-CBT is marginally superior to Eye Movement Desensitisation and Reprocessing (EMDR). There is also a substantial literature demonstrating its effectiveness in the treatment of complex trauma (The Complex Trauma Taskforce 2012; Briere and Scott 2015).
>
> There have been no controlled trials of psychological therapies for PTSD in people with intellectual disabilities. But there is evidence that adaptations of TF-CBT are effective with children (e.g. Gillies et al. 2015), and there is evidence from other indications such as anger and depression that adults with intellectual disabilities who have mental health problems can benefit from adapted CBT group interventions (Vereenhooge and Langdon 2013; Willner and Lindsay 2016).
>
> Positive effects of CBT-based interventions have been reported in case studies of people with intellectual disabilities with PTSD (Willner 2004; Stenfert Kroese and Thomas 2006) and a review of this literature concludes that 'evidence based methods have to be developed to treat people with various levels of ID who suffer from PTSD. A first step might be to systematically evaluate the use of already established methods such as trauma-focused CBT' (Mevissen and De Jongh 2010).

Many of the themes we identified when we analysed the interview data provided by the clients who took part in TF-CBT groups overlap with the studies mentioned earlier. For example, 'being listened to' and being in the presence of other people who also experienced trauma in the past is described as helpful although some clients had had initial misgivings about joining such a group:

> One good thing is you get to meet different people. It's nice to know you're not by yourself, that other people have had things happen in their life too.

On the other hand, people also reported that being a member of a therapeutic group can be challenging and emotionally painful and that identifying with other group members is difficult. So it is important that CBT therapists carefully consider the pros and cons of group versus individual therapy for each of their clients. Some people may not yet have the resilience, motivation or confidence to function in a therapeutic group.

People who took part in the TF-CBT groups also talked about the cost of having to share the time and attention that therapists are able to devote to each client:

> Sometimes it was quite difficult because they when they [other group members] were anxious they obviously talk a lot (laughs) and so … staff were focussing all their attention on them and so we found it a bit difficult because obviously we couldn't really get a word in edgeways.

This client also reports that, unlike fellow group members, she did not enjoy the relaxation exercises with which every group session ended, yet endured this part of the session for the sake of the others:

> I know a lot of the people like the relaxation at the end but I didn't like it very much because I don't find it very easy to relax so when they were sat there with their eyes closed I was thinking, 'this is weird.' (laughs) I can't deal with that very well, but yeah.

Some clients chose to be accompanied by a support worker in order to deal with the stress of being in a group setting. This worked well for a number of people who otherwise would not have attended the group sessions.

One client points out how difficult it was for him to talk about his problems and to listen to other people's problems. He also reports that having a support worker present was helpful and that his anxiety reduced with time:

> Sometimes I had to push myself to go ... It was stressing me out sometimes talking about different subjects ... At the time it made me anxious but towards the end I coped a bit better, the right support helped. If I'd gone on my own [without a support worker] then it wouldn't have worked. Certain things were hard to talk about. I remember the way [group therapist] didn't load too many questions on, that helped, because I was a bit worried discussing in front of everyone else. It felt a bit stressful when others were talking about certain things.

But the presence of support workers also has potential disadvantages:

> I didn't like the men in the group, the carers. They reminded me of the bad experiences I've had.

This client found the presence of male support workers disturbing as the past trauma she had experienced was perpetrated by male staff. She raised an important issue relating to the common theme of 'feeling safe in the group'. As all clients who attend our TF-CBT groups have experienced severely traumatising events in their past, their evaluation of the group is often phrased in terms of how safe they feel in that setting. Most clients comment on this in a positive way, for example:

> Knowing you could go talking to people you could trust.

They report that they have benefited from the intervention in terms of improved mental health, ability to cope with PTSD symptoms and being able to share their problems. For example:

> I'm still nervous around new people, but I talk more than I did. My attitude has changed, before I didn't talk much but now I open up to talk more.

Some comment that positive change occurred gradually:

> It's harder at the beginning then towards the end you can see some light at the end of the tunnel. I've been in a lot of places before where I felt there weren't no light at the end of the tunnel.

They also allude to the importance of needing further support in their daily life to maintain these benefits:

> Yes, I know the techniques to cope. I took away the 'soles of the feet' [mindfulness exercise], I still do that, I've got my mom on to it as well because it helps.

The aspects of the group intervention these clients remember best and rate most highly are role play and relaxation exercises, and therapists taking part in the exercises:

> And they (staff) joined in as well, which was good fun. Knowing that they're listening. Because you can tell that they're interested as well in the past and what's been going on 'cause they're doing it with you, they're not sitting on it even though they're listening they're actually doing it with you, which was really great.

As in previous studies, it was the shared social experiences and developing positive relationships with the therapists and other group members that people responded most positively to, rather than specific elements of the CBT intervention. While individual CBT interventions may offer opportunities to form an exclusive therapeutic relationship and to communicate openly and in-depth with the therapist, they cannot provide the same forum for social support and the development of multiple and sometimes lasting relationships. It seems from what our clients tell us that the group itself is perceived as an important vehicle for therapeutic change. This is important when considering the context in which most of our clients experience psychological problems. When our clients talk about what causes them distress and trauma and what triggers their anger, they usually talk about difficulties associated with relationships. Similarly, the examples they give of having used recommended coping strategies are typically embedded in situations involving relationships and interactions with other people. So, given that relationships appear a key source of distress, provocation, but also of support and encouragement, the provision of a group-based intervention addresses their problems head on by providing opportunities to discuss and rehearse coping strategies in a social context, and also opportunities to experience positive relationships, even when discussing difficult subject matter. This brings us neatly back to the Marsh quote used at the beginning of this chapter: 'By the crowd they have been broken, by the crowd they shall be healed.'

The underlying message of this quote has implications that extend beyond the delivery of psychological therapies to more general aspects of service provision for people with intellectual disabilities. Clients' appreciation of open discussion and the development of positive relationships is strikingly present in all of the qualitative studies on group therapy for people with intellectual disabilities. It is our experience that in their day-to-day lives, opportunities to speak about themselves and their emotions, and to form meaningful relationships with the people around them, are limited. There could be considerable benefits (not only for those with mental health problems) if health and social services were to consider ways in which their service users might be offered more opportunities to simply talk and be listened to. Also, giving a clear message from an early age onwards that experiencing difficult feelings such as sadness, anger, fear and jealousy is universal and unavoidable, and that recognising and dealing with these emotions involve skills that can be learned and can often avoid further distress for self and others, is likely to prevent mental health problems in later life. Psycho-educational programmes for children such as 'Zippy's Friends' (Mishara and Bale 2004; see box below) have a good evidence base (e.g. Holen et al. 2012) and a version of 'Zippy's Friends' adapted for Special Needs Schools has recently been evaluated (Unwin and Stenfert Kroese 2015).

> Zippy's Friends is a school-based mental health promotion programme that aims to teach social, emotional, problem-solving and coping skills to help children develop strategies to deal with difficult social situations and help them feel better about such situations while at the same time avoiding harm to others and themselves. The focus is on the development of emotional literacy and it takes a solution-focused approach to emphasise positive emotions, strengths and sources of support. The six modules cover a range of topics: emotions, communication, friendships and dealing with change and loss. We consider such an early group intervention approach to equip children with ID with coping skills and the awareness that talking about difficult feelings can be helpful, an excellent preventative strategy for a population at high risk of developing mental health problems.

Some Considerations

What follows now are some considerations for therapists who are interested in delivering CBT in a group setting. Although the aims of your group may be different from the ones that we have run, we hope that with our experience of CBT group work and the useful feedback from our clients, we can pass on some general tips and ideas for future CBT group work with people with intellectual disabilities. For a more detailed guide to group work, although not specific to our client group, we recommend Holmes's (2010) 'Psychology in the real world—community-based group work' which is a detailed and honest account of many relevant theoretical and practical aspects and issues, reporting on successes as well as some eye-watering failures.

Preparation

A particular challenge to group dynamics can result from clients moving from 1:1 therapy to group work with the same therapist. Although sometimes unavoidable, we have found that this can present problems. Because the client is used to having the full attention of the therapist and is not used to sharing this with others, it makes it more difficult for them to enter into dialogue and identify with the group, and we would avoid this if at all possible.

When you and your colleagues are planning a group, make sure that you let other people know that you are recruiting and advertise your group in clear and positive terms. We have found that sometimes our groups are perceived as useful time fillers for people who are receiving very few other services but don't really need psychological therapy. We have also found that some staff give clients the impression that they have to attend the group because they have been 'bad' or need 'sorting out', something you may be able to avoid by stressing the voluntary and constructive nature of your group in your information leaflets and posters.

Having a decent venue with space, light and easy access is a priority. Many health and social services buildings now have doors that require a security code to enter and exit. This can make some clients feel very uncomfortable (particularly when they feel they can't leave the building) so if you are unable to avoid them, make sure you explain the need for these security measures and discuss ways in which group members can indicate that they want to leave and feel as relaxed as possible about this.

We also pay attention to the quality of drinks and biscuits we offer to people in break times, the stationary and art materials we use (good quality and age-appropriate), and the way in which people are welcomed into the building and into the therapy room. Therapists should greet everyone by name and introduce people to each other. All these small details can have a significant impact on the way in which clients perceive their group membership, their self-esteem and the importance placed on continued attendance.

Meet clients individually before you offer them a place in the group. This allows you to obtain their informed consent (make clear what the group entails, its purpose and aims and the pros and cons of CBT group work) as well as establishing what clients' aims are, what they hope to get out of attending the group. We use a measure developed in Shropshire (see www.toolsfortalking.wordpress.com) that we have found to be a quick and easy way to start talking about people's personal goals. You can also ask them to complete (with your help) any psychometric measures that can help you to evaluate the overall efficacy of the group (pre-post and ideally follow-up measures). But make sure you explain the reasons why you are asking them all these questions as some clients may experience this as intrusive. For example, one member of a TF-CBT group (Stenfert Kroese et al. 2016) stated:

The downside is the questions you get asked, I know they ask everyone but I'm not like that. Like the ones asking have you been violent towards others, they can make you feel uncomfortable because I've not been brought up like that. I don't like questions like that, it makes me feel intimidated, and you're the victim, you aren't the violent one.

Group Identity

Because we want people to feel that they belong to a group that they can be proud of and feel a part of, it is important to think of a positive and catchy title. For example, when a few years ago we received a number of referrals for people with anger problems we advertised the upcoming group as 'Dealing with difficult feelings' group rather than 'Anger Management' group so as to avoid the labelling of group members as 'angry people'. One of the key messages that we wanted to convey is that anger is a universal emotion which everyone will experience at times and which need not be suppressed but can be expressed in a way that is constructive and not harmful for self or others. This will also improve the chances of self-referrals rather than clients being 'sent' (unwillingly?) by others, which can only be good for motivation and group dynamics.

We record a lot of the work we do in the group sessions on flip chart sheets that can be blue tacked on the walls. Digital photographs of these are then taken at the end of the session, printed and given out as hand-outs at the beginning of the next session, to be added to each person's folder. If they are able to use their phone to take and store photos, then clients can collate them electronically and they can serve as 'on the spot' prompts in their daily lives. Whether paper or electronic, we have found that these records function as memory aids and create a sense of ownership of the materials and information shared within the group. This adds value to the work group members do and gives them an opportunity to reflect on the contributions they made in previous sessions, which can have a positive impact on their confidence and motivation to take part in further group activities.

Making the Group Accessible and Safe

For some people, being in a group setting will be anxiety provoking and they may need plenty of reassurance and support both before and during the group sessions. For some people it is comforting to have a support worker or other familiar person with them at all times. For others it may be enough to have someone with them for just the first session, after which they feel safe enough to come on their own.

Sometimes it will be important to have gender-specific groups especially when clients have experienced abuse from perpetrators of the opposite sex. As is the case for all therapy work, when organising groups we operate under a number of constraints and exclusively male, female (or other gender variations) groups may not always be possible although with a well-established rolling programme of group work within a large catchment area, it may be easier to organise more homogeneous group membership.

Likewise, with unlimited resources and venues, locations that are accessible and feel safe and not too clinical in appearance are preferred, but in reality we may have to compromise. What then becomes important is that the clients are supported not just by the group therapists but also by the important people in their home environment. We also recommend that you communicate with the receptionists and other staff who the clients may encounter and give them sufficient information so they are aware of your clients' specific needs and can be a welcoming, helpful and reassuring first port of call when people enter and exit the building.

Some clients may not feel comfortable closing their eyes during the relaxation exercises and then following an easy read script can act as a useful focus point. This can help some clients to take part in the exercise and remain engaged for the duration so they don't disrupt the quiet and relaxing atmosphere. Another way to engage these clients may be to offer them music or text that they can listen to through earphones.

Support Staff

During screening sessions discuss with group members whether they would like to have a support person with them and who this person could be. We have had friends, family (including someone's grandmother) and support staff come along and many of them have been not just supportive to the client but also helpful and contributing to the rest of the group. But make it clear that a consistent family member or staff allows for a 'closed' group and offers a safer environment in which people can share difficult feelings and experiences than when the group has to be introduced to a different support person every week. Because of staff rotas and shortages, achieving this consistency is not always possible. We have had five different members of staff supporting one client over the course of a group. To compensate for this, we made sure that each new support worker was introduced to the group, a brief summary of the aims and rules of the group was given to them and they were asked to participate in all activities. Although there are obvious constraints to guaranteeing consistent attendance, negotiation at the screening stage, preferably with service managers, may avoid the disruptive impact of frequently introducing new members into the group.

We expect therapists as well as support staff to fully participate in the group activities and to complete, for example, their own Hassle Logs (anger management diaries) to discuss within the group. Staff talking through their own Hassle Logs may help clients become more confident in completing and reporting their own logs. Also, by openly sharing our own anger problems with group members, they may become aware that most people struggle at times with their feelings and that difficult feelings can be expressed in constructive ways.

Through supporting an individual in the group, a worker can gain a better understanding of the person they support, and the presence of staff can significantly improve the long-term outcomes of group interventions (Rose et al. 2005). Staff can become more informed about the reasons why an individual may react in a situation and so can more easily externalise the attribution of blame rather than blaming the person with the intellectual disability (who may be unable to communicate the reasons behind their actions). Also, by staff becoming more psychologically minded, their knowledge is likely to generalise to how they work with other people they support and ultimately influence their practice in a wider context.

We have found that the presence of support staff can be helpful for some of the group members and allows them to attend and feel safe and supported during the sessions.

Also, because we have to cater for the varying needs of group participants due to different communication and literacy skills levels and attention span, having extra staff allows for greater flexibility. For example, with able and willing support staff you can break into small groups to accommodate participants' different needs and offer more support to the less able clients with reporting back on diaries and other tasks and exercises. Another scenario where support staff can be helpful is when a group member becomes distracted or disengages. A client fell asleep a couple of times during one of our CBT groups. We were able to deal with this by assigning a support worker to him so he could take a break from the group if needed.

However, there were a number of disadvantages to the attendance of support staff. It made one service user feel unsafe (see above) and it sometimes affected the continuity of the group when different support staff accompanied the client for each group session. Unfortunately, we have also found that some support staff can act inappropriately, belittling their clients, undermining their confidence or disclosing confidential information. In one case, this worrying behaviour resulted in one of the group therapists meeting with the manager of a service and as a result of this conversation, a one-day staff-training event around clients' psychological needs was offered. We now strongly recommend that, before accompanying a client to one of our groups, support staff are asked to attend a brief training session so that they are aware of the ethical and psychological principles on which the group intervention is based. We also ask managers to allocate the same support worker throughout the course of the group intervention in order to avoid undue disruption to the group dynamics.

Enforcement of Group Rules

In all of our CBT groups we make sure that group rules are agreed during the first session. We write them on a flip chart that is blue tacked on the wall at every session and referred to frequently. Sometimes people struggle to adhere to the rules and the group therapists need to think carefully how to address this without seeming to be overbearing or patronising. During one group, a client who lived alone and came to the group on his bicycle was consistently late. In order to aid his memory and help him with time management, one of the group therapists would ring him one hour before the agreed starting time of 10 a.m. This improved his punctuality and reduced the disruption caused by his late arrival, without us having to resort to mentioning his lateness (and that he was breaking the group rules) in front of other group members. At other times, a discussion about how not adhering to the rules may affect the group can be useful, for example, when a member of the group frequently interrupts.

In one of our groups, a client repeatedly spoke about an argument she had had with her mother, which began to irritate other group members. This client could not read the subtle cues emanating from facilitators and clients alike and when more directive strategies were used she became overly apologetic and we were concerned that she might feel upset about being publically 'corrected'. So we tried to 'open up' the discussion to other group members when this client was talking at length (e.g. 'Has anyone else had problems with family?') before moving on to the next agenda item. We also decided that as facilitators we would place particular emphasis on the group agenda, agreeing on a tight list on a flip chart at the outset and repeatedly returning to the list during sessions. We then always referred to the agenda when anyone 'hogged the floor' and stressed to the whole group that we needed to move on. We normalised this as being a group rule that applied to clients as well as facilitators. Not a perfect solution but it worked to some extent.

Cognitive Strategies

Our clients are usually able to recall several of the behavioural components of the intervention at follow up but often no cognitive coping skills are recalled spontaneously, although with prompting usually people remember them. These components are more difficult to convey and so perhaps less well understood or at least less well remembered and thus less frequently implemented in daily life. It is therefore important to find ways in which the cognitive strategies are most effectively presented during the group sessions and the feedback from clients has provided us with some realistic and practical suggestions. For example, over the years we have introduced more role play and other 'doing' activities (such as art work and quizzes) as well as DVD clips, and the information imparted during each session is presented in smaller 'chunks'. Other authors agree that in group work for adults with intellectual disabilities 'procedures should be oriented more towards activity than discussion' (Razza and Tomasulo 2005).

The role play activities provide opportunities for the group to 'bring to life' personally relevant situations. It not only allows group members to think about situations they find difficult to handle but as therapists we can gain deeper insight and we can support group members with problem solving on how to adopt alternative (adaptive) strategies. One technique we have found effective is using a remote TV control to 'freeze' the role players in their tracks at crucial moments. This allows the therapist to ask the relevant player about their thoughts and feelings and linking these with past and future events. Pressing the 'play' button allows the role play to continue.

Peer Support

We have observed that some group members prefer to act with each other in their role play scenarios rather than with therapists and yet others feel safer when a therapist joins in. We would encourage therapists to consider the huge benefits of peer support and peer relationships and try to use every possible opportunity to encourage our clients to interact with each other during group activities. When this happens spontaneously, we sacrifice the 'agenda' and allow the discussion to move away from the planned session content to encourage group members to share their experiences and to advise, encourage and empathise with each other. In this way, relationships can sometimes develop within the group that may continue 'post intervention'. For example, in one 'Dealing with difficult feelings' group, two men continued to see each other after the group finished and supported each other to join a local men's group.

Endings and Then?

As in 1:1 therapy, we need to make sure that our clients are aware of the time-limited nature of the intervention and remind them regularly of how many sessions have taken place and how many are still to come. We have found it helpful to ask group members to plan how they want to spend the last session or at least the end part of that session. Often people appreciate the chance to celebrate their achievements and enjoy a fairly formal ceremony involving cake and the handing out of attendance and achievement certificates.

We also arrange a follow-up session approximately three months after the last session so that people can tell each other and us how they have been able to maintain and generalise the progress they have made and how they are coping. We have already mentioned how important peer relationships are and how powerful peer support can be and we therefore also encourage people to continue to meet with each other in non-clinical settings.

Nevertheless, our qualitative research on group interventions indicates that clients as well as staff have difficulties maintaining and generalising successful coping strategies in 'real life' and in the long term. Retaining improved psychological well-being without support is difficult for our clients and encouragement and support from other adults in their immediate environment is without doubt crucial for long-term positive outcomes. As with 1:1 CBT interventions, we recommend that group therapists ensure that for each client who has taken part in the group, at least one reliable person (whether staff, family or friend) is recruited and trained in providing such long-term support after the group sessions have ended.

> **Key Points**
> - CBT group work has been shown to be beneficial for people with intellectual disabilities and feedback from clients suggests that the *non-specific effects* of the group intervention are particularly valued. We therefore consider the influence of other psychological approaches such as systemic, interpersonal, person-centred and psychodynamic therapies as complementing our CBT interventions.

- Being listened to and being taken seriously by therapists and other group members is often mentioned as a positive and unusual experience by our clients, suggesting that this is a service deficiency that if addressed could prevent or at least ameliorate mental distress and mental health problems.
- When offering CBT group therapy, attention must be paid to preparation and practical issues such as how to advertise and recruit, how to choose and prepare the venue, and how to assess the clients' psychological needs and goals.
- Making the group accessible, comfortable and safe, and encouraging a positive group identity are important aspects to consider and can improve attendance and reduce dropout.
- Having support staff or family members accompany the clients and take an active part in the group can have both advantages and disadvantages and needs to be carefully planned.
- How best to enforce group rules and how to end the group in a way that maximises the chances that progress is maintained in the long term must also be considered at an early stage.

References

Bender, M., & Tombs, D. (1992). How should we measure the effect of groupwork with adults with learning difficulties? I. Outcome variables. *Clinical Psychology Forum, 43*, 2–6.

Bisson, J. L., Roberts, N. P., Andrew, M., Cooper, R., & Lewis, C. (2013) Psychological therapies for chronic post-traumatic stress disorder (PTSD) in adults. *The Cochrane Library*, Issue 12. Art. No.: CD003388. DOI: 10.1002/14651858.CD003388.pub4.

Briere, J., & Scott, C. (2015). Complex trauma in adolescents and adults: Effects and treatment. *Psychiatric Clinics of North America, 38*(3), 515–527.

British Psychological Society, Royal College of Psychiatrists and Royal College of Speech and Language Therapists. (2007). *Challenging behaviour: A unified approach*. Leicester: British Psychological Society. http://dcp-ld.bps.org.uk/document-downloadarea/document-download$

Braun, V., & Clarke, V. (2006). Using thematic analysis in psychology. *Qualitative Research in Psychology, 3*(2), 77–101.

Gillies, D., Taylor, F., Gray, C., O'Brien, L., & D'Abrew, N. (2015). Psychological therapies for the treatment of post-traumatic stress disorder in children and adolescents. *Evidence Based Child Health, 8*, 1004–1016.

Halgin, R. P. (1985). Teaching integration of psychotherapy models to beginning therapists. *Psychotherapy: Theory, Research, Practice, Training, 22*(3), 555–563.

Holen, S., Waaktaar, T., Lervag, A., & Ystgaard, M. (2012). The effectiveness of a universal school-based programme on coping and mental health: A randomised, controlled study of Zippy's friends. *Educational Psychology, 32*(5), 657–677.

Holmes, G. (2010). *Psychology in the real world – Community-based groupwork.* Ross-on-Wye: PCCS Books.

Marsh, L. C. (1953). *Group treatment of the psychoses.* http://www.metro.inter.edu/facultad/esthumanisticos/coleccion_anton_boisen

McLeod, J. (2011). *Qualitative research in counselling and psychotherapy (2nd ed.).* London: Sage.

MacMahon, P., Stenfert Kroese, B., Jahoda, A., Stimpson, A., Rose, N., Rose, J., Townson, J., Hood, K., & Willner, P. (2015). 'It's made all of us bond since that course…' – A qualitative study of service users' experiences of a CBT anger management group intervention. *Journal of Intellectual Disability Research, 59*(4), 342–352.

Mevissen, L., & de Jongh, A. (2010). PTSD and its treatment in people with intellectual disabilities: A review of the literature. *Clinical Psychology Review, 30*, 308–316.

Mishara, B., & Bale, C. (2004). An international programme to develop the coping skills of six and seven year old children. In S. Saxena & P. Garrison (Eds.), *Mental health promotion from countries: A joint publication of the world federation for mental health and the world health organisation.* WHO Library Cataloguing-in-Publication Data.

Novaco, R. W. (2003). *The Novaco anger scale and provocation inventory (NAS-PI).* Los Angeles: Western Psychological Services.

Pert, C., Jahoda, A., Stenfert Kroese, B., Trower, P., Dagnan, D., & Selkirk, M. (2013). Cognitive behavioural therapy from the perspective of clients with mild intellectual disabilities: A qualitative investigation of process issues. *Journal of Intellectual Disability Research, 57*(4), 359–369.

Razza, N. J., & Tomasulo, D. J. (2005). *Healing trauma: The power of group treatment for people with intellectual disabilities.* Washington, DC: American Psychological Association.

Rose, J., Loftus, M., Flint, B., & Carey, L. (2005). Factors associated with the efficacy of a group intervention for anger in people with intellectual disabilities. *British Journal of Clinical Psychology, 44*(3), 305–317.

Smith, J. A., Flowers, P., & Larkin, M. (2009). *Interpretive phenomenological analysis: Theory, method and research*. London: Sage.

Stenfert Kroese, B., & Thomas, G. (2006). Treating chronic nightmares of sexual assault survivors with an intellectual disability – Two descriptive case studies. *Journal of Applied Research in Intellectual Disabilities, 19*, 73–80.

Stenfert Kroese, B., Gillott, A., & Atkinson, V. (1998). Consumers with intellectual disabilities as service evaluators. *Journal of Applied Research in Intellectual Disabilities, 11*(2), 116–128.

Stenfert Kroese, B., Willott, S., Taylor, F., Smith, P., Graham, R., Rutter, T., Stott, A., & Willner, P. (2016). Trauma-focussed cognitive-behaviour therapy for people with mild intellectual disabilities: Outcomes of a pilot study. *Advances in Mental Health and Intellectual Disabilities, 10*(5), 299–310.

The Complex Trauma Taskforce. (2012). The ISTSS expert consensus treatment guidelines for complex PTSD in adults. www.istss.org/AM/Template.cfm?Section¼ISTSS_Complex_PTSD_Treatment_Guidelines&Template¼%2FCM%2FContentDisplay.cfm&ContentID¼5185. Accessed 7 Nov 2016.

Unwin, G., & Stenfert Kroese, B. (2015). *An independent evaluation of Zippy's friends for children and young people with special educational needs* (Final report for the Judith Trust). http://www.partnershipforchildren.org.uk/uploads/File/Evaluation_Zippys_Friends_Judith%20Trust.pdf

Vereenhooge, L., & Langdon, P. E. (2013). Psychological therapies for people with intellectual disabilities: A systematic review and meta-analysis. *Research in Developmental Disabilities, 34*, 4085–4102.

Vos, T., Haby, M. M., Magnus, A., et al. (2005). Assessing cost-effectiveness in mental health; helping policy-makers prioritize and plan health services. *Australian and New Zealand Journal of Psychiatry, 39*, 701–712.

Whitfield, G. (2010). Group cognitive-behavioural therapy for anxiety and depression. *Advances in Psychiatric Treatment, 16*(3), 219–227.

Whittington, A., & Grey, N. (2014). *How to become a more effective CBT therapist -mastering metacompetence in clinical practice*. Oxford: Wiley Blackwell.

Willner, P. (2004). Brief cognitive therapy of nightmares and post-traumatic ruminations in a man with a learning disability. *The British Journal of Clinical Psychology, 11*, 222–232.

Willner, P. (2015). The neurobiology of aggression: Implications for the pharmacotherapy of aggressive challenging behaviour by people with intellectual disabilities. *Journal of Intellectual Disability Research, 59*(1), 82–92.

Willner, P., & Lindsay, W. R. (2016). Cognitive behaviour therapy. In N. Singh (Ed.), *Clinical handbook of evidence-based practices for individuals with intellectual disabilities*. Cham: Springer.

Willner, P., Rose, J., Jahoda, A., Stenfert Kroese, B., Felce, D., Cohen, D., MacMahon, P., Stimpson, A., Rose, N., Gillespie, D., Shead, J., Lammie, C., Woodgate, C., Townson, J., Nuttall, J., & Hood, K. (2013). Group-based cognitive-behavioural anger management for people with mild to moderate intellectual disabilities: Cluster randomised controlled trial. *The British Journal of Psychiatry, 203*(4), 288–296.

Yalom, I. D., & Leszcz, M. (2005). *The theory and practice of group psychotherapy* (5th ed.). New York: Basic Books.

9

Mindfulness and Third Wave Therapies

In the opening chapters of this book we highlighted the long-standing health inequalities faced by people with intellectual disabilities, in particular their limited access to talking therapies. Whilst we hope that the provision of accessible CBT signifies some progress on this front, the push for greater equity is an ongoing process. Therapies naturally evolve and develop over time and we must keep up with the changing landscape to ensure that clients with intellectual disabilities don't get left behind. Over the past ten years or so new trends in therapy have been particularly evident with the rapidly growing interest in emerging 'third wave' therapies such as Mindfulness Based Cognitive Therapy (MBCT), Compassion Focused Therapy (CFT) (Gilbert 2009), Acceptance and Commitment Therapy (Hayes et al. 1999) and Dialectical Behaviour Therapy (Linehan 1993). Despite having much in common with standard CBT, a key difference is that third wave therapies tend to target the process of thoughts, rather than engaging with the content, and usually place a strong emphasis on the mind body connection.

In this chapter we will consider what this new brand of therapies may have to offer clients with intellectual disabilities, focusing predominantly on mindfulness-based interventions. We consider how the core principles of mindfulness differ from that of CBT and discuss some challenges that might be faced when using mindfulness with clients who have an intellectual disability. We will end with some consideration of adaptations that may improve accessibility.

Mindfulness in Health Settings

Mindfulness-based approaches are now widely offered in health services throughout the UK, Europe and the USA. In the National Health Service in the UK, an eight-week group-based programme is commonly offered, with weekly sessions of between two and three hours' duration. Sessions typically involve a taught psycho-educational component, guided group mindfulness exercises, a CD of guided mindfulness meditations to facilitate home-based practice, and a half-day or full-day silent mindfulness retreat.

Jon Kabat-Zinn first introduced mindfulness into the health care system in the USA in the 1990s when he developed Mindfulness Based Stress Reduction (MBSR) for patients suffering chronic pain (Kabat-Zinn 1990, 1994). Inspired by this innovation, a group of clinicians and researchers working on the prevention of relapse in depression collaborated with Kabat-Zinn and went on to develop MBCT which has an added CBT component (Segal et al. 2002). The surge in popularity for MBCT, which followed publication of the seminal book *Mindfulness Based Cognitive Therapy for Depression*, has continued to gather momentum, leading to a second edition of the book being published in 2013 (Segal et al. 2013).

The endorsement of mindfulness-based interventions within the National Health Service context has to a large extent been driven by growing evidence of the benefits of this approach for a range of health problems (including pain, HIV and AIDS, cancer) and mental health and well-being, including depression and anxiety (for a review see Khoury et al. 2013). There is a strong body of evidence showing the benefits of MBCT for people suffering from depression, including individuals who have experienced more than three relapses of depression (Teasdale et al. 2002; Ma and Teasdale, 2004; Kuyken et al. 2008, 2012; Williams et al. 2014). This research led to mindfulness being recommended by the National Institute for Health and Care Excellence in England and Wales (NICE) as an evidence-based intervention and Scottish Intercollegiate Guidelines Network guidelines (NICE 2009; SIGN 2010). Another body of literature looking at the benefits of mindfulness for cognitive control suggests that mindfulness is associated with improved selective attention, working memory and aspects of executive function such as emotion regulation and self-regulation of behaviour, attracting interest within education settings.

Mindfulness and People with Intellectual Disabilities: What's the Evidence?

There is a small body of research exploring adapted mindfulness interventions for clients with an intellectual disability, as well as other diverse groups such as older adults, children and people with acquired brain injury (Bedard et al. 2005, 2012; Azulay et al. 2013; Flook et al. 2013). The majority of studies in the intellectual disabilities field have explored the benefits for carers who support people with intellectual disabilities, where encouraging benefits have been found using both mindfulness approaches and Acceptance and Commitment Therapy (Singh et al. 2006, 2015; Noone and Hastings 2010).

A recent review paper by Harper et al. (2013) identified 18 studies where mindfulness was offered to clients with intellectual disabilities or their paid carers. Notably, carer studies were included only if the outcomes measured were client related (e.g. client behaviour change). The review included four studies where other third wave therapies such as Acceptance and Commitment Therapy and Dialectical Behaviour Therapy were used. Mostly, the research focused on observed changes in aggressive behaviour. Twelve of the studies were carried out by one research group led by Nirbhay Singh. Ten studies showed evidence of reduced client aggression and five studies showed improved emotional well-being, including evidence of reductions in stress, depression and obsessive thoughts. Other benefits highlighted by the same review are increases in pro-social behaviour, staff satisfaction, parenting satisfaction, levels of happiness (perceived), social functioning and a reduction in staff sick leave.

The growing body of research showing the potential benefits of using mindfulness with carers offers great encouragement; however, in this chapter we aim to focus on developments in mindfulness for people who have an intellectual disability. As things stand, the evidence that this is a helpful therapy for people with intellectual disabilities is limited, with most research consisting of single case studies using an adapted mindfulness technique called 'meditation on the soles of the feet' developed by Nirbhay Singh and colleagues. This approach teaches clients to shift their attention from the precursors of emotion such as anger, to their body, specifically the soles of the feet. The use of role play in sessions offers the person a clear context and rationale for practising the body awareness technique. This approach will be described in more detail later in this chapter when considering adaptations for people with intellectual disabilities.

One published study to date has sought to adapt the eight-week MBCT programme for clients with intellectual disabilities (Idusohan-Moizer et al. 2015). Again, the 'meditation on the soles of the feet' technique was used by the facilitators, alongside a mindfulness of breathing meditation and exercises focusing on compassion. The group participants were offered ten sessions with a follow-up session six weeks later. The study found that participants showed a reduction in anxiety, depression, improved self-compassion and compassion for others. Another study by Chapman and Mitchell (2013) explored the views of individuals with an intellectual disability who attended an introductory workshop on mindfulness, which also involved a short meditation practice. Participants responded favourably saying that mindfulness could be a helpful way to cope with emotional difficulties. A recent study by Clapton et al. (2017) explored the feasibility of adapting a CFT group for people with a mild intellectual disability. Six participants took part in the adapted six-week group programme. The findings showed that all participants were able to engage with compassion exercises, and that CFT groups specifically adapted for adults with mild intellectual disabilities are feasible and acceptable for this client group. The authors suggest that further adaptations to the CFT group structure and content, such as increasing the number of sessions, would be beneficial.

So What Is Mindfulness?

We don't set out to offer an in-depth account of mindfulness here, and would refer the reader to a number of excellent resources that are available (Kabat-Zinn 1990, 1994; Crane 2008; Segal et al. 2002, 2013). Rebecca Crane provides a helpful, concise summary of the theoretical underpinnings in her book *Mindfulness Based Cognitive Therapy*, describing the key components of the MBCT programme session by session.

The most widely quoted definition of mindfulness is 'paying attention in a particular way: on purpose, in the present moment, and non-judgmentally' (Kabat-Zinn 1994). Shauna Shapiro emphasises three core qualities of mindfulness: (a) present-centred attention and awareness, (b) intention or purposefulness, which highlights a motivational component to one's attention and behaviour, and (c) attitude, which reflects how we attend, or the qualities that one brings to the act of paying attention, such as interest, curiosity, non-judgement, acceptance, compassion and receptiveness (Shapiro et al. 2006).

Mindfulness: A Different Process

Perhaps one of the most striking differences between CBT and MBCT is the largely experiential route taken in mindfulness sessions. In MBCT each session begins and ends with a mindfulness practice, with a further mindfulness exercise of at least 30 minutes duration during the group. The exercises most commonly used in MBCT are described briefly below.

> **MBCT Mindfulness Exercises**
>
> Mindfulness of Breathing. In this exercise the breath is used as a focus for the attention during a sitting meditation, usually lasting approximately 30 minutes. Concentrating solely on the breath encourages a focus on the present moment. Participants become more aware of the natural tendency of their mind to wander and can practise refocusing their attention on the breath.
>
> Mindfulness of Eating. In this exercise, also referred to as the 'raisin exercise', participants are given a raisin and encouraged to explore the sensory experience with a 'beginner's mind', as though they have never seen, held or tasted a raisin before. The exercise encourages the individual to recognise that the experience of eating can be transformed by paying attention in this way.
>
> Body Scan. In the body scan participants focus their attention on each part of the body in turn and simply notice whatever sensations they are experiencing. Participants are encouraged to bring an attitude of curiosity, acceptance and kindness to the experience. Body awareness encourages participants to notice the changing sensations in the body and offers a different vantage point into the emotional states that are experienced.
>
> Mindful Movement. The practice of mindful movement involves attending to the physical sensations of the body whilst engaged in a sequence of movements, usually involving stretching and balancing. Participants are encouraged to tune in to the changing bodily sensations, whilst recognising the limits of their body and noticing mental states such as striving for particular results or self-criticism.

There is an established set of learning objectives for each MBCT group session, which are conveyed using experiential and didactic methods. The session plan across the eight weeks is:

1. Awareness and autopilot.
2. Living in our heads.
3. Gathering the scattered mind.
4. Recognising aversion.
5. Allowing and letting be.
6. Thoughts are not facts.
7. How can I best take care of myself.
8. Maintaining and extending new learning.

A combination of mindfulness practices and facilitated discussion (called the inquiry process), allows the mindfulness facilitator to convey the key principles of non-judgement, patience, the beginner's mind, trust, acceptance, non-striving and letting go. A full overview of the specific learning points embedded in the various mindfulness exercises can be found in the Bangor, Exeter and Oxford Mindfulness Based Interventions Teaching Assessment Criteria (MBI-TAC), (Crane et al. 2012). These include learning to be fully with experience; learning to see recurring patterns in the mind; relating skilfully to the mind wandering and refocusing; noticing and relating to body sensations; experiencing the difference between automatic pilot and present moment awareness.

Mind and Body

In mindfulness there is strong emphasis on developing body awareness. As there is less demand on verbal skills, body awareness exercises can be a good option, or a helpful starting point, for people with intellectual disabilities. Also, the physical sensations of the body can act as an indirect route to better emotional understanding, as the early signs of mood change are often most easily observed in our body. By practising the body scan exercise in particular (see above), clients can develop a greater awareness of the physical cues that reveal their emotional state. This can in turn lead to a heightened sense of control over emotions in everyday life and an anchor point back into the present moment.

In their recent book, Paul Gilbert and Choden (2014) also point to the benefits of 'grounding in the body' when in difficult circumstances. Grounding techniques can help prevent clients from getting caught up in the narratives attached to the surrounding situation. The soles of the feet are a good place to start as a grounding technique; feeling the connection to the ground or floor encourages a sense of stability. This is in keeping with the 'meditation on soles of the feet' approach for people with intellectual disabilities (Singh et al. 2007), which also teaches clients to focus on the soles of their feet as a way of diverting attention from emotionally arousing thoughts or experiences. When practising grounding techniques, Gilbert and Choden propose practising a second 'compassion' element, of turning an attitude of kindness and compassion to felt physical sensations.

Mindfulness: A Different Relationship with Your Problems

Whereas most emotion regulation strategies aim to change the nature of emotions by re-evaluating the situation or suppressing the emotion through distraction or some other means, mindfulness encourages people to observe their emotional experiences without trying to change them. In mindfulness the instruction is to accept experiences, and let go of the tendency to label one's emotions as good or bad. The emphasis is on noticing the natural habits of the mind and accepting difficulties as an inevitable part of life experienced by us all, to a greater or lesser extent. In our own clinical work we have found that normalising problems can have particular value for people with intellectual disabilities, as a socially marginalised and stigmatised group who often experience a sense of inadequacy and failure. This is a strong advantage of mindfulness. As the aim is not to 'fix' problems, there is no implicit assumption that those participating are 'broken' in some way. The non-judgemental attitude adopted in mindfulness *embraces* difference and moves people away from self-blame and criticism. A sense of equality is reinforced by the full participation of facilitators in the programme, and discussion about their own mindfulness practice. The process neither pathologises nor medicalises problems; indeed, the fact that there is no focus on a diagnosed 'problem' during mindfulness sessions is in line with stance taken by the British Psychological Society Division of Clinical Psychology (BPS-DCP) regarding clinical diagnosis in mental health.

Key mindfulness principles of awareness and acceptance also encourage an entirely different way of relating to difficulties. With the practice of present moment awareness, participants are encouraged to simply be aware of whatever is happening as it is happening. This is the central learning point covered in the first four sessions of the MBCT programme. By focusing attention on the present moment there is a realisation that often we are operating on automatic pilot, preoccupied by our own internal dialogue. This typically involves either thinking about the past or worrying about the future. Either way, the problem is that we continue to be 'there' rather than 'here'. The benefit of present moment awareness during times of difficulty is that awareness allows us to step back from our experience and distance ourselves, at least to some extent, from the narrative that we habitually attach to problems. Intentional awareness on the present moment encourages us to become more focused on aspects of experience *other* than the problem.

However, despite the suggested benefits of present moment awareness, it's not easy to focus our attention in the here and now. Often we don't feel in control of our thoughts, and our mind naturally jumps around or gets stuck on things that are distressing or worrying. As mentioned, the foundational skill practised to develop awareness is to place the attention on a chosen object or sensation, notice when the mind wanders and repeatedly bring the mind back. This is an ongoing process and there is no expectation that the mind will stop wandering. However, with practice it is expected that we can become more aware of the habits of the mind and become better at refocusing the attention. This is the main objective of Singh's soles of the feet meditation adapted for people with intellectual disabilities. Some techniques that we have found helpful when supporting people with intellectual disabilities with this practice are discussed later in this chapter.

Those practising mindfulness are encouraged to turn *towards* difficulties with curiosity and acceptance, which is a stark shift from the usual habit of avoidance or pushing against problems. This is perhaps the aspect of mindfulness that is most counterintuitive and challenging for practitioners. Yet, paradoxically, the notion that it's okay to feel bad can be quite a relief to many clients. We found this to be the case when running a drop-in mindfulness group, which we called the 'How Do I Feel Group', for people with intellectual disabilities. The slogans 'We all have good days and bad days' and 'Everyone gets stressed, it's a normal part of life' became popular catchphrases for many participants. The process of accepting difficulties as simply being part of everyone's wider experience rather than indicating failure seemed to go some way to reduce a sense of inferiority and alienation from others. This could be an important benefit of mindfulness for people with intellectual disabilities, as these are often the very concerns that underpin anxiety problems or low mood.

We should clarify that acceptance doesn't mean giving up or letting others treat you badly. On the contrary, it is more akin to the validation of all feelings, both positive and negative. The truth is that when we try to escape unpleasant emotions (experiential avoidance), this can reinforce unhelpful assumptions, meaning that these thoughts and feelings become strengthened. The basis of acceptance is to recognise that difficult emotions are an inevitable part of life and therefore can't fully be avoided no matter how hard we struggle against them. Indeed, it is argued that we can actually endure our difficult emotions more easily if we don't expect that things should or can be otherwise. The notion of simply accepting that you are anxious, rather than resisting and pushing against it, has similar underpinnings to the work addressing metacognitive difficulties (Wells 2007). CBT therapists are well aware that it is often the clients' cognitions *about* their emotional difficulties that exacerbate their distress (e.g. anxious thoughts about being anxious). In fact, these metacognitive difficulties are often the main focus of CBT work. In mindfulness the notion is that strategies aimed at escaping unpleasant thoughts and feelings can reinforce unhelpful assumptions, just like experiential avoidance, meaning that these tend to come back even stronger. Dan Siegel points out that the expectation that we should be constantly at ease or happy can actually lead to much disappointment and unhappiness, leading us to get caught up in distressing thoughts about how things 'should' be, which simply adds to our distress. So, with mindfulness skills, we can begin to recognise that our usual focus on 'this is how it should be' is at times part of the problem, and that accepting 'this is how it is' will reduce our distress (Siegel 2007). Rebecca Crane comments:

> We come to see that the best way of achieving our goals is often to back off from striving for results and to start seeing and accepting things as they are. (Crane 2008)

In a clinical setting, the practice of acceptance can also improve participants' ability to *tolerate* negative emotional states and to cope with them more effectively, recognising that distressing experiences cannot necessarily be avoided or resolved (Baer 2003).

Acceptance: Paradoxes inherent in the process of acceptance
Learning to be at ease with not feeling at ease
Letting go of the struggle to change and fix ourselves makes change more likely

Mindfulness: A Different Relationship with Your Thoughts

In CBT the main focus is on noticing unhelpful thought patterns and reconstructing these. Mindfulness also teaches greater awareness of thoughts, but encourages us to notice, acknowledge and be curious about our thoughts without trying to change them and without getting caught up in the storyline. This isn't the same as rejecting thoughts; rather, it involves stepping back, or 'decentring', from thoughts. By decentring in this way, and staying in the present moment, it's possible to gradually overcome the mind's tendency to rerun events from the past. Whilst this is by no means an easy task, it could offer a helpful alternative for clients with intellectual disabilities who may not be able to reconstruct or reframe their thoughts. When people are unable to shift perspective, then a decentring element can be introduced to facilitate loosening their grip on the thought loop. This offers one example of how mindfulness can be used in conjunction with other more established CBT methods, to make them more effective. When using thought decentring techniques there is no need to elicit alternative thoughts to replace unhelpful thinking, meaning that these techniques can be applied broadly across a range of circumstances. The decentring approach also lends itself well to the use of visual imagery and active techniques such as physically letting thoughts go. Singh et al. (2011) used a similar technique with people with an intellectual disability, using the metaphor of thoughts being like clouds drifting through the sky. We discuss below how the decentring technique was adapted for use with one client to overcome her problems of anxiety.

Case Example

Anne is a 26-year-old woman with a mild intellectual disability, referred due to long-standing anxiety problems, mainly involving social anxiety. She had become increasingly anxious since beginning a new college course, due to her concerns about socialising with the other students. She lacked confidence when meeting new people and due to her anxiety avoided sitting with other students at the break. She was convinced that her classmates noticed how uncomfortable and awkward she was feeling, and felt humiliated. She would avoid talking in the class for fear that she might say something 'stupid' and make a fool of herself. She experienced unhelpful thoughts of inadequacy and ridicule such as 'I am sad and useless' and 'they think I'm an idiot'.

A decentring technique was introduced following unsuccessful attempts to use cognitive restructuring techniques in sessions. Anne was unable to shift perspective and continued to believe that her anxious thoughts were accurate. Before introducing decentring techniques some groundwork was needed. Firstly, Anne was introduced to the notion of the 'busy mind' using a mindfulness exercise where she was encouraged to simply notice any thoughts that passed through her mind. This helped Anne to notice that even when she was doing nothing her mind was busy with thoughts. The 'busy mind' was normalised, as was the experience of anxious thoughts passing through the mind. Secondly, Anne was encouraged to tune in to her thoughts at ten-minute intervals during one session. This demonstrated to Anne that her thoughts were constantly changing, even within a short period of time, and that thoughts naturally come and go of their own accord with no effort required. The learning objective of this exercise was to reduce Anne's belief that she couldn't escape from anxious thoughts. Given the transient nature of thoughts, as demonstrated during the exercise, their perceived 'importance' was challenged. Taken together, these two building blocks offered a basis for the decentring technique.

Anne was then encouraged to practise letting her anxious thoughts 'drift off into the distance', using the image of letting go of a balloon. She personalised the image choosing her favourite colour and used a cue card with this image (see below) to remind her to use the technique when she noticed anxious thoughts.

Anne practised using the 'Let it go' technique whilst travelling on the bus to college, when she noticed anxious thoughts or had a 'busy mind'. She reported benefits, such as a greater sense of control over her anxiety and a greater tolerance of social settings. Yet, whilst Anne benefitted from the thought distancing technique, she retained a wish to reject distressing or anxious thoughts. As is the case with many clients, she found the concept of acceptance of thoughts considerably more difficult than letting them go.

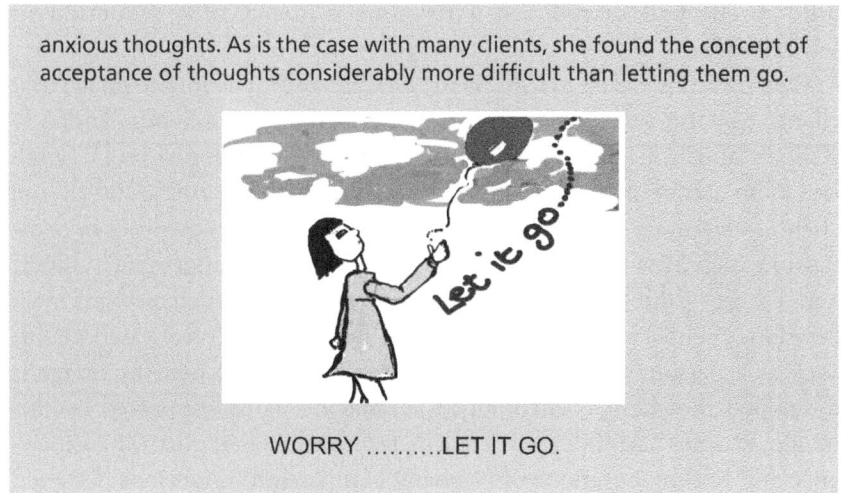

WORRY ....LET IT GO.

A Different Relationship with Yourself: Using Compassion

Following from the mindfulness principle of acceptance comes an attitude of self-acceptance and kindness towards yourself. In MBCT this compassion component is not explicit, but rather is embedded in the process of the exercises and inquiry process, where qualities of self-compassion and self-acceptance are encouraged and modelled by the mindfulness facilitator. In CFT, compassion is more central to the process and is explored in the context of an evolutionary 'three-systems' model comprising the 'threat' system (focused on dangers), 'drive' system (orientated towards achievement) and 'affiliative soothing system' (involving a sense of safeness and feelings of interpersonal connectedness). Gilbert proposes that people with early chaotic relationships, trauma and shame can have an overactivated threat system and a less functional soothing system. The emphasis in CFT is on helping clients to develop and activate the soothing system. As mentioned earlier, a recent feasibility study by Clapton et al. (2017) showed promising results using an adapted CFT group approach with participants with mild intellectual disabilities, with some evidence of a reduction in self-criticism.

One technique used in CFT is to cultivate a compassionate image that clients can use to connect with a sense of comfort, safeness and care (Gilbert and Irons 2004). This exercise has been developed by Deborah Lee to be used with clients suffering from trauma (Lee 2005, 2009). The client is encouraged to develop an image that embodies qualities of compassion such as wisdom, strength, warmth and non-judgement (Gilbert and Proctor 2006). As the compassionate image is each person's own creation, clients can use any source that helps them to feel cared about, such as a person, animal or an image from nature. When the image is developed the client is encouraged to imagine being supported by this image, at times of difficulty to 'tune in' to the associated nurturing experience and bodily sensations of receiving compassion. Questions designed by Gilbert and Proctor (2006) to help clients develop their compassionate image are shown below.

Building a compassionate image
How would you like your ideal caring compassionate image to look?
How would you like your ideal caring compassionate image to sound (e.g. voice tone)?
How would you like your ideal caring compassionate image to relate to you?
What other sensory qualities can you give to it?
How would you like your compassionate image to relate to you?
How would you like to relate to your ideal caring-compassionate image?

Taken from Gilbert and Proctor (2006)

Later in this chapter we suggest ways of adapting the compassionate image exercise for people with intellectual disabilities.

Kristin Neff and Chris Germer (2012) have developed a range of self-compassion strategies in their work. Neff points out that self-compassion is not based on positive evaluations of ourselves (like self-esteem), but rather is a way of *relating* to ourselves in times of difficulty. Instead of attacking and berating ourselves for being inadequate, self-compassion techniques can be used to actively self-soothe by offering ourselves warmth, encouragement and acceptance. As the actual felt quality of these experiences can be difficult to express in words it is helpful to encourage clients to tune into an awareness of the associated physical sensations.

For clients, such as those with an intellectual disability, who commonly have concerns about being different or lacking social status, the compassionate stance promoted in CFT and mindfulness could have particular benefits, if adaptations are made to the process.

Ways of Adapting Mindfulness

Alongside the need to adhere to an evidence-based mindfulness approach, there is also recognition of the need to adapt mindfulness to meet the specific needs of different groups. Jon Kabat Zinn has said:

> We emphasize that there are many different ways to structure and deliver mindfulness-based stress reduction programs. The optimal form and its delivery will depend critically on local factors and on the level of experience and understanding of the people undertaking the teaching. (Jon Kabat-Zinn 1996)

Many of the ideas we have previously suggested for adapting CBT can equally be applied to mindfulness and other third wave therapies. Common difficulties relating to communication, attention and memory can be addressed by keeping exercises short, providing more repetition and using visual aids. As mentioned earlier in this chapter, Singh et al. (2007) have made substantial adaptations to the usual process and content of mindfulness exercises in their soles of the feet meditation, This approach uses a more guided, instructional style than traditional mindfulness techniques, and has a specific focus on increasing awareness and attentional control. The trainers' manual published by the authors (Singh et al. 2011) gives clear and specific guidelines for the practitioner to follow, including techniques that are used to support clients to tune in to emotional experiences and shift their attention. Ten training steps are outlined which involve eliciting emotion and then shifting the attention from these emotional events to the body (soles of the feet).

Keep It Real: Making Sense of Abstract Concepts

One challenge for those practising, as well as those teaching, mindfulness is that many of the key concepts are fairly intangible and abstract. This can be off-putting for many people new to mindfulness and certainly represents a challenge when working with clients who have intellectual disabilities. Linehan (1993) has considered ways to make the key concepts more accessible when using Dialectical Behaviour Therapy, an approach she developed specifically for people who have enduring and complex needs. When working with people who may have difficulty grasping the underlying principles, it is generally advised that the therapist 'starts small', breaking down the definition of mindfulness into the key concepts and translating these into context, spelling out how these might apply in situations the person finds difficult in real life rather than talking in the abstract. We will discuss other ways of making mindfulness relevant later in this section.

Generally, mindfulness facilitators make use of CDs and hand-outs to support learning and encourage practice in between sessions. However, clients with intellectual disabilities will generally require a more individualised approach to reflect each person's particular needs. When running a mindfulness drop-in group we gave clients personal mindfulness packs, using materials thought to be most suitable for each individual, such as photographs of themselves practising movement postures, their favourite sensory objects, cue cards with relevant learning points, mindfulness of music CDs and photographs of comfort images. Some clients added photographs of their favourite happy memories. The packs proved helpful for participants and also offered a resource for carers to help them reinforce learning points and support home practice. In a study carried out with people who had acquired brain injury, connections between learning activities were made more explicit by asking that participants record their observations and questions on forms they called 'new learning' forms, to encourage deeper reflection (Bedard et al. 2003). For clients with intellectual disabilities, we have found the use of cue cards to capture ideas relating to the key principles of mindfulness has served a similar function (see below). These phrases can then be recorded on flip charts as 'catch-phrases' or slogans to be repeated in future sessions and copied for clients to incorporate into their pack of materials. Examples of some catch-phrases are 'It's good to slow down and focus'; 'Everyone gets upset at times – that's just part of life'; 'We all have good days and bad days'; 'When things are difficult it helps to be kind to ourselves.'

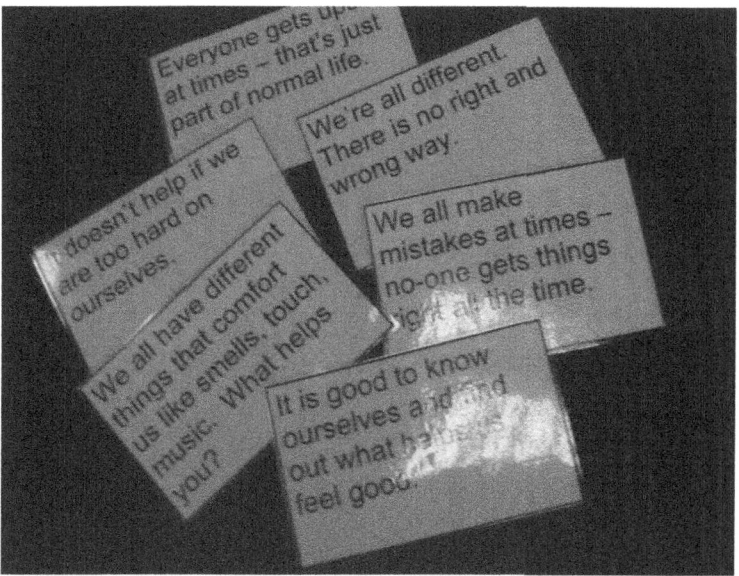

As the purpose of mindfulness exercises can be somewhat obscure, the link between the exercises practised during sessions and the potential benefits in everyday life should be made explicit when working with people with an intellectual disability. One option is to offer clients an initial awareness session in advance of the group, where the basic principles and benefits of practising mindfulness can be presented in layman's terms. Mindfulness online programmes, such as MindUp, devised specifically for children have used this approach, often with pre-mindfulness teaching about how stress affects the body and mind, and how mindfulness can help. Similar educational preparatory work has been used with individuals who have acquired brain injury (Bedard et al. 2013).

Making Mindfulness Relevant

Singh et al. (2007) used role play to support clients' learning and establish clear goals when using mindfulness techniques to deal with problems of anger control. They suggest a range of role plays that can be used within sessions, such as responding to someone who is saying something that offends you; responding to a peer who is threatening to hit you; responding to a staff member or co-worker who is not nice to you; responding to someone who pushes you around.

Another way of illustrating mindfulness principles, and showing how these apply in real life, is to use a storyboard approach. We have used stories to present common 'unmindful' habits (such as operating on automatic pilot), compared with a 'mindful' alternative. Stories can be supported with a series of photographs or line drawings in the same way described in Chap. 4. An example of a mindfulness storyboard script is shown below together with the group discussion points used to reinforce the key principles.

Storyboard: Automatic pilot versus awareness
1. <u>Automatic pilot</u> Billy is at the swimming pool. While he is swimming Billy is thinking about all the things he has to do later that day. He begins to worry that he won't have enough time. His mind is caught up in thinking about how he can get things done. He rushes to finish his swimming session. He doesn't notice that his friend has come into the pool. <u>Group discussion points</u> • What is Billy paying attention to when swimming? • Is he enjoying it? • Does he notice what's happening around him? 2. <u>Practising present moment awareness</u> The next time Billy goes to the swimming pool he practises keeping his mind on swimming. He takes things *slowly* so that he can take it all in. He pays attention to the smell of the pool, and notices the warm feeling of the water against his skin. He notices the noises in the pool and the colour of the water. When his mind drifts he brings it back and focuses on how it feels to be swimming <u>Group discussion points</u> • What is different for Billy this time? • What is Billy paying attention to when swimming? • Is he enjoying it? • Does he notice what's happening around him? • What are the benefits of focusing on the present moment?

Storyboards can also be used to explore self-criticism versus self-compassion or ruminating versus decentring from thoughts. As well as using this approach to improve understanding of the principles of mindfulness, we have found that the learning objectives are understood and remembered more easily and are more likely to be translated into real life. This was shown to be the case when after using this approach one group member told us that she had advised her brother to 'slow down' when he was rushing his meal, suggesting that our automatic pilot story had resonated.

Make It Easy: Engaging People with Intellectual Disabilities in Mindfulness

Mindfulness requires practice and persistence, and there is always a risk that clients will give up too quickly before experiencing the benefits. Judson Brewer discusses common difficulties faced by people new to mindfulness and suggests that it is helpful to start with positive experiences, such as tuning into a pleasant sensory object (Brewer et al. 2013), as it is easier to bring a sense of curiosity and beginner's mind to something we enjoy. This offers a greater incentive to continue, and acts as a stepping stone to the more traditional exercises. Similarly, Singh and colleagues also suggest an initial focus on a 'happy' situation in their manual (Singh et al. 2011). Following the same principle, we have found that using sensory-focused exercises is an engaging and enjoyable starting point for clients with intellectual disabilities. We have encouraged clients to explore smells, touch, sounds, colours and shapes, using a sensory box with items such as hand cream, smooth stones, soft fabric, sparkling objects, bubble wrap and music. The process of sensory awareness exercises follows the same learning points as those explored in the mindful eating exercise, tuning in and adopting an attitude of curiosity then discussing the experience with group members. Sensory exercises can also show that we all have different preferences—and that's okay.

We have found that mindfulness exercises that involve sitting and paying attention to the breath can prove challenging for many clients with an intellectual disability. Some clients become easily distracted, perhaps because the breath doesn't provide a clear anchor for the attention. Other clients have a tendency to try too hard, taking exaggerated, effortful breaths. In line with this, Salzberg and Goldstein (2001) suggest that rather than beginning with the breath, those new to meditation should start with a focus on sounds, simply bringing attention to any sounds that can be heard in the room. In line with this we found that an exercise in mindful listening using music as a focus point was a popular starting point for clients with intellectual disabilities, and worked well for those who were less comfortable sitting in silence. Another option for mindful listening is a group game involving participants listening to recognisable sounds such as a bird singing, a baby crying, laughter, a car engine. The group can take turns to describe what they hear.

Awareness of emotions can be encouraged by exercises involving tuning into how we feel. We have started groups with a short discussion of how group members are feeling NOW (this minute) and then tracked this on a feelings thermometer 0–10 before and after mindfulness exercises. By avoiding the tendency to label emotions as being either good or bad, the facilitator can model the acceptance of feelings, and point out the habit of trying to 'fix' negative feelings.

The Problem of the Wandering Mind

In mindfulness, the tendency for the mind to wander is accepted as a normal habit of the mind, experienced by everyone to a greater or lesser degree. Nevertheless, it might be assumed that people with intellectual disabilities will be more susceptible to difficulties on this front. Some clients with intellectual disabilities will struggle to engage with the basic requirements of mindfulness exercises that require sitting still, staying quiet and persisting with something that is difficult. Firstly, it should be remembered that mindfulness doesn't only involve sitting meditation exercises and clients can choose to stick with more 'active' exercises, such as mindful eating and mindful movement.

Nevertheless, it would be easy to conclude that mindfulness is simply not suitable for clients with intellectual disabilities due to their poor attention control. But a growing research literature shows convincing evidence of the beneficial effects of mindfulness training *to enhance cognitive control* such as improved cognitive flexibility (Moore and Malinowski 2009), improved attentional processing (Chambers et al. 2008; Tang et al. 2007; Jha et al. 2007), the ability to inhibit impulsive responses and improved self-regulation (Teper and Inzlicht 2013). This raises the possibility that people with intellectual disabilities stand to gain *even more* from mindfulness due to their common difficulties with attention and self-regulation. Whilst this is clearly speculative, some support for the notion is offered by a recent study carried out with children. Flook et al. (2010) introduced mindfulness training in a school classroom and compared the benefits for children with poor executive function (and poor behaviour regulation) and those without such problems. The findings suggested greater benefits for the children who had executive function difficulties. This would be an interesting area for future research.

For clients with an intellectual disability who have problems of poor attention and distractibility, a more guided approach can be used. It can also be helpful to break into smaller groups for some exercises. For instance, when doing mindful movement the facilitator needs to tailor their approach according to the varying physical abilities of each participant. Or when practising mindfulness of breathing, where the objectives of the exercise are less clear, the facilitator might use active techniques to support clients who become distracted. In some cases this might include verbally prompting a client who has lost focus by quietly and gently pointing this out to them. By acknowledging the distraction, in a non-judgemental and supportive manner, the facilitator may gradually increase the client's insight and awareness. Usually the prompt in itself is enough for the person to re-engage with the exercise. The facilitator can simply reassure the person that it's okay and normal for this to happen; then prompt them to refocus in their own time. As noted earlier, the meditation on soles of the feet (e.g. Singh et al. 2011) offers similar, guided instruction on refocusing the attention. We have also used visual cues such as placing coloured stickers on the feet to offer a visual prompt to help clients refocus their attention on the soles of the feet.

Keep It Short and Repeat Often

Similar to CBT, a slower pace and more repetition of information during sessions will be helpful to overcome problems of attention and memory. For instance, mindfulness exercises can be shortened to take account of attention problems, but repeated more often during the course of sessions, to build familiarity and understanding. It might be better to practise two short exercises rather than one more lengthy version. A similar adaptation was shown to be effective in a study carried out with people who had acquired brain injury; the eight-week MBCT course was extended to ten sessions and practice sessions were shortened (Bedard et al. 2014; Flook et al. 2013).

Working with Compassion

When working with clients with intellectual disabilities, it can be difficult to find appropriate words to represent the concept of compassion. Once again, stories and role play can be used, such as stories about someone being kind to you, listening to you, sticking up for you, forgiving you. For more able clients we have adapted the compassionate image exercise described earlier. An example is described below:

> **Case Example: Using a Compassionate Image**
>
> Mary was referred with problems of anger, low mood and verbal aggression towards members of her staff team. She has a mild intellectual disability and cerebral palsy. She receives support from a social care organisation four hours each day within her own home.
>
> Mary had a disrupted early childhood and spent frequent spells in foster care. She has ongoing difficulty sustaining relationships and worries about being unpopular or being a burden to others. She describes herself as unlikeable and anticipates that she will be rejected by others and be left on her own and lonely. Mary has also shown a tendency to idealise others, often leading to a breakdown in the relationship when she feels let down or rejected. She has a history of conflict with social care staff, describing

some staff members as being too bossy and critical. She often refuses to let members of her support team into her home, which then heightens her fears about being left on her own. She describes strong physiological symptoms such as an empty feeling in her stomach and chest.

Building Blocks

Before using the compassionate image exercise, some preparatory work was necessary. Grounding techniques were introduced to help Mary feel more in control of her physiological symptoms. Then photographs depicting acts of compassion (such as one person consoling another and someone tending to a sick animal) were used to encourage Mary to tune in to the feelings that these images stimulated.

A compassionate image exercise adapted to suit Mary's needs was introduced. Adaptations included (i) simplification of terminology, (ii) a more guided approach, such as the therapist suggesting the 'kind words' which might be spoken, (iii) using photographs from magazines and drawings to help develop a visual image, (iv) setting clear homework tasks to encourage Mary to practise the technique in real life.

Initially, when developing her compassionate image, Mary struggled to imagine an image that would fit this role. She was asked to imagine: 'Someone who is kind; cares about you; gives you good advice; Someone who understands how you feel and doesn't judge you.' Mary was encouraged to choose any image that would work for her, including a person, animal or object from nature. Despite her initial difficulty developing her own image, Mary's demeanour during the exercise suggested she was engaged with the exercise, so we agreed that it was worth persisting.

Initially the main focus was placed on identifying 'kind words' that Mary would find comforting at times of distress, rather than on the visual image. She was able to choose from compassion statements suggested by the therapist (such as 'I'll always be here for you; I understand how you feel; I'll take care of you'). Mary then went on to develop a visual image that she called her 'comfort cat'. This image was based on a pet cat Mary had looked after when younger. She described a physical sense of ease and relief associated with her comfort cat image ('warm, like I'm floating'). Interestingly, she described this as a relationship where she and the comfort cat cared about and looked after each other. Notably, reciprocal relationships had been lacking in her life. Despite a slow start, Mary went on to develop her compassionate image, doing homework prior to sessions for the first time, such as developing a script using photographs to represent the comfort cat image supported by her carer (see below).

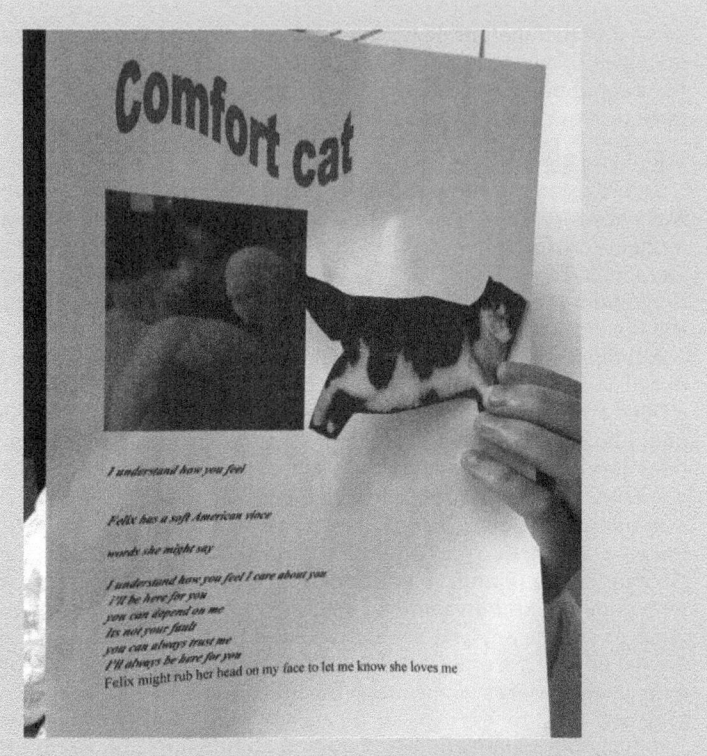

Some improvements were shown in Mary's ability to regulate her emotions and in her ability to cope with setbacks. Opposition towards her staff team reduced and she was generally found to be more accepting of support. The positive impact of the compassionate image exercise was evident during one session when Mary spoke about an interaction she had with a sales assistant earlier that week. This had been a relatively fleeting interaction but left a strong impression on Mary, who commented on the sales assistant's patience and kind attitude, and described an associated sense of connection and validation. It seemed unlikely that this brief encounter would have been so salient, or beneficial, prior to Mary's work using the compassionate image.

The compassionate image exercise won't be suitable for all clients and other compassion techniques can be tried, such as encouraging clients to think about, and 'tune in' to a time when they felt safe or cared about. Photographs depicting images of kindness, affection and nurturing can also be used as a helpful springboard to discuss the feelings associated with compassion. Photographs of happy memories can be used to recall a sense of connection with loved ones. Caution is clearly required when working with clients who have had disrupted early relationships or traumatic experiences, to ensure that the task is not distressing. An exercise involving discussion of memories of receiving kindness can be incorporated into a group and acted out in role play. Group members have told us that they are comforted by someone listening, having company, talking about problems, getting a cuddle, a hug. Often clients find it difficult to find the words to describe these compassion-based feelings, in which case it is best to introduce this as an experiential rather than verbal exercise. It can be helpful to encourage 'tuning in' to the physical sense experienced when looking at photographs that elicit a sense of care and kindness. As usual the therapist can offer initial guidance if required, by suggesting options (e.g. you might notice a warm, fluttery feeling in the chest, soft stomach, tingling sensation.)

Adapting Mindfulness to Suit Different Physical Needs

Many clients with intellectual disabilities have problems with balance and coordination, or physical limitations such as impaired function of their legs or arms, which could affect their ability to engage with movement exercises. In order to ensure safety the facilitators should gather information regarding physical difficulties beforehand and in some cases specialist advice should be sought to ensure that active movement exercises are suitable. Movement exercises can be adjusted for those who prefer to sit on a chair or use a wheelchair, as the same process of tuning in to body sensations can be achieved when sitting or standing. For clients who require more individualised support due to physical needs it may be best to have additional facilitators to allow personal support when needed. Similar adaptations have been used for older adults (Zellner et al. 2014).

Some clients may find it difficult to sit still, or sit comfortably in which case it can help to use props to reduce discomfort. People of small stature can use a small raised block to rest their feet more comfortably. Other clients might like to hold a small cushion or soft ball during sitting meditation to offer a focus point and reduce restlessness. As mentioned earlier it is likely that shorter practice exercises will work best.

Practising at Home

Maintaining regular home practice is a well-recognised challenge for most people practising mindfulness, and can pose a particular challenge for those with an intellectual disability, especially those who have difficulties with planning and organisation. In such cases, adaptations similar to those suggested in previous chapters might be helpful, such as setting concrete tasks and agreeing on a specific time and place to practise. In some cases practical difficulties can present a barrier to home practice. One client who lived in shared accommodation told us she found it difficult to find a quiet space to practise mindfulness and another client didn't have access to technology to listen to guided CDs. Involving carers in mindfulness sessions can increase their awareness and encourage them to support home practice.

Mindfulness Isn't for Everyone

As with any new approach there is a need for caution. A few recent papers have highlighted concerns that researchers in the mindfulness field generally fail to explore or monitor potential adverse effects of the approach (e.g. Dobkin et al. 2012). Lustyk et al. (2009) provide a review of adverse effects that may be experienced, including psychological and physical negative effects. They conclude that participants should be screened carefully before being offered mindfulness. Similarly, Marshall and Holmes (2009) recommend that mindfulness groups should have two facilitators so that any problems that may arise for more vulnerable participants can be dealt with effectively. As such, it is important that future research considering the potential benefits of mindfulness for people with intellectual disabilities should also take account of possible adverse effects and contraindications.

Conclusions

There is a keen interest in developing mindfulness for people who have intellectual disabilities. The work of Singh and colleagues (e.g. Singh 2007) has shown encouraging outcomes using an adapted mindfulness intervention, soles of the feet meditation. We have discussed some adaptations that may improve the accessibility of standard mindfulness programmes such as the MBCT eight-week programme. Yet we should not confine the approach too narrowly. Mindfulness needs to be engaging for people with an intellectual disability, who may have limited persistence and low tolerance for a process that takes time to show effects. As mindfulness grows in popularity, new creative ideas are emerging, such as incorporating mindfulness with the arts, music and the outdoors. Some of these innovations might be particularly applicable for clients with an intellectual disability, perhaps more so than the standard mindfulness approaches.

We hope that future research will also explore the effectiveness of other third wave therapies, such as CFT, which we believe may hold real promise for people with intellectual disabilities.

Key Points
1. Mindfulness exercises lend themselves well to adaptations, allowing each person to find exercises that suit their preference and abilities.
2. Many of the adaptations we have suggested for mindfulness are in line with those used for CBT, such as keeping exercises short, providing more repetition and using visual aids and storyboards to overcome communication difficulties.
3. Other adaptations are more specific to the mindfulness model, including the need to clarify abstract concepts and support clients to interpret and apply the key principles of mindfulness.
4. Mindfulness needs to be engaging for clients with an intellectual disability, who may otherwise have limited persistence.

5. Alongside adaptation of the eight-week MBCT for use with clients who have a learning disability, a range of other creative methods should be explored.
6. More research is required to explore the benefits and key ingredients of mindfulness for clients with an intellectual disability.

References

Azulay, J., Smart, C. M., Mott, T., & Cicerone, K. D. (2013). A pilot study examining the effect of mindfulness-based stress reduction on symptoms of chronic mild traumatic brain injury/postconcussive syndrome. *Journal of Head Trauma Rehabilitation, 28*(4), 323–331.

Baer, R. A. (2003). Mindfulness training as a clinical intervention: A conceptual and empirical review. *Clinical Psychology, 10*, 125–143.

Bédard, M., Felteau, M., Gibbons, C., Klein, R., Mazmanian, D., Fedyk, K., & Mack, G. (2005). A mindfulness-based intervention to improve quality of life among individuals who sustained traumatic brain injuries: One-year follow-up. *Journal of Cognitive Rehabilitation, 23*, 8–13.

Bédard, M., Felteau, M., Marshall, S., Gibbons, C., Klein, R., & Weaver, B. (2012). Mindfulness-based cognitive therapy: Benefits in reducing depression following a traumatic brain injury. *Advances in Mind-Body Medicine, 26*, 14–20.

Bedard, M., Felteau, M., Marshall, S., Cullen, N., Gibbons, C., Dubois, S., Maxwell, H., Mazmanian, D., Weaver, B., Rees, L., Gainer, R., Klein, R., & Moustgaard, A. (2014). Mindfulness-based cognitive therapy reduces symptoms of depression in people with a traumatic brain injury: Results from a randomized controlled trial. *The Journal of Head Trauma Rehabilitation, 29*, 13-22.

Brewer, J. A., Davis, J. H., & Goldstein, J. (2013). Why is it so hard to pay attention, or is it? Mindfulness, the factors of awakening and reward-based learning'. *Mindfulness, 4*, 75–80.

Chambers, R., Lo, B. C., & Allen, N. B. (2008). The impact of intensive mindfulness training on attentional control, cognitive style, and affect. *Cognitive Therapy and Research, 32*, 303–322.

Chapman, M. J., & Mitchell, D. (2013). Mindfully valuing people now: An evaluation of introduction to mindfulness workshops for people with intellectual disabilities. *Mindfulness*. doi:10.1007/s12671-012-0183-5.

Clapton, N., Williams, J., Griffith, G., & Jones, R. (2017). Finding the person you really are … on the inside. *Journal of Intellectual Disabilities, Jan 1*, 1744629516688581.

Crane, R. (2008). *Mindfulness-based cognitive therapy: Distinctive features*. Routledge: Taylor and Francis.

Crane, R. S., Soulsby, J.D., Kuyken, W., Williams, J.M.G., Eames, C. (2012). *Bangor, Exeter and Oxford mindfulness based interventions teaching assessment criteria (MBI-TAC)*. Centre for Mindfulness Research and Practice, School of Psychology, Bangor University.

Dobkin, P. L., Irving, J. A., & Amar, S. (2012). For whom may participation in a mindfulness-based stress reduction program be contraindicated? *Mindfulness, 3*(1), 40–44.

Flook, L., Kitel, M., Kaiser-Greenland, S., Locke, J., Ishijima, E., & Kasari, C. (2010). Effects of mindfulness awareness practices on executive functions in elementary school children. *Journal of Applied School Psychology, 26*, 70–95.

Flook, L., Goldberg, S. B., Pinger, L., Bonus, K., & Davidson, R. J. (2013). Mindfulness for teachers: A pilot study to assess effects on stress, burnout and teaching efficacy. *Mind, Brain and Education, 7*, 182–195.

Gilbert, P. (2009). Introducing compassion-focused therapy. *Advances in Psychiatric Treatment, 15*(3), 199–208.

Gilbert, P. (2010). *The compassionate mind. Compassion focused therapy*. London: Constable and Robinson.

Gilbert, P., & Choden, K. (2014). *Mindful compassion. How the science of compassion can help you understand your emotions, live in the present, and connect deeply with others*. Oakland: New Harbinger Publications.

Gilbert, P., & Irons, C. (2004). A pilot exploration of the use of compassionate images in a group of self-critical people. *Memory, 12*(4), 507–516.

Gilbert, P., & Proctor, S. (2006). Compassionate mind training for people with high shame and self-criticism: Overview and pilot study of a group therapy approach. *Clinical Psychology and Psychotherapy, 13*, 353–379.

Harper, S., Webb, T., & Rayner, K. (2013). The effectiveness of mindfulness-based interventions for supporting people with intellectual disabilities: A narrative review. *Behaviour Modification, 3*, 431–453.

Hayes, S. C., Strosahl, K. D., & Wilson, K. G. (1999). *Acceptance and commitment therapy: An experimental approach to behaviour change*. New York: Guildford Press.

Idusohan-Moizer, H., Sawicka, A., Dendle, J., & Albany, M. (2015). Mindfulness-based cognitive therapy for adults with intellectual disabilities: An evaluation of the effectiveness of mindfulness in reducing symptoms of depression and anxiety. *Journal of Intellectual Disability Research, 59*(2), 93–104.

Jha, A. P., Krompinger, J., & Baime, M. J. (2007). Mindfulness training modifies subsystems of attention. *Cognitive Affective Behaviour Neuroscience, 7*, 109–119.

Kabat-Zinn, J. (1990). *Full catastrophe living: Using the wisdom of your body and mind to face stress, pain and illness*. New York: Delta.

Kabat-Zinn, J. (1994). *Wherever you go, there you are: Mindfulness meditation in everyday life* (p. 4). New York: Hyperion.

Kabat-Zinn, J. (1996). Mindfulness meditation: What it is, what it isn't, and its role in health care and medicine. In Y. Haruki, Y. Ishii, & M. Suzuki (Eds.), *Comparative and psychological study on meditation*. Delft: Eburon.

Khoury, B., Lecomte, T., Fortin, G., Masse, M., Therien, P., Bouchard, V., Chapleau, M. A., Paquin, K., & Hofmann, S. G. (2013). Mindfulness-based therapy: A comprehensive meta-analysis. *Clinical Psychology Review, 33*(6), 763–771.

Kuyken, W., Byford, S., & Taylor, R. S. (2008). Mindfulness-based cognitive therapy to prevent relapse in recurrent depression. *Journal of Consulting Clinical Psychology, 76*, 966–978.

Kuyken, W., Crane, R., & Dalgleish, T. (2012). Does mindfulness based cognitive therapy prevent relapse of depression? *British Medical Journal, 345*, e7194. doi:10.1136/bmj.e7194.

Lee, D. A. (2005). The perfect nurturer: Using imagery to develop compassion within the context of cognitive therapy. In P. Gilbert (Ed.), *Compassion: Conceptualisations, research and use in psychotherapy*. London: Brunner-Routledge.

Lee, D. A. (2009). Using a compassionate mind to enhance the effectiveness of cognitive therapy for people who suffer from shame and self. In D. Sookman & R. Leahy (Eds.), *Treatment resistant anxiety disorders*. New York: Routledge.

Linehan, M. (1993). *Cognitive behavioural treatment of borderline personality disorder*. New York: Guilford Press.

Lustyk, M., Chawla, N., Nolan, R., & Marlatt, G. (2009). Mindfulness meditation research: Issues of participant screening, safety procedures, and researcher training. *Advances in Mind Body Medicine, 24*(1), 20–30.

Ma, S. H., & Teasdale, J. D. (2004). Mindfulness-based cognitive therapy for depression: Replication and exploration of differential relapse prevention effects. *Journal of Consulting Clinical Psychology, 72*, 31–40.

Marshall, M., & Holmes, G. (2009). An evaluation of a mindfulness group. *Group, 19*, 40–58.

Moore, A., & Malinowski, P. (2009). Meditation, mindfulness and cognitive flexibility. *Conscious Cognition, 18*(1), 176–186.

National Institute for Health and Clinical Excellence. (2009). *Depression: The treatment and management of depression in adults (update)*. Clinical Guideline 90, p. 34. London: NICE.

Neff, K. D., & Germer, C. K. (2012). A pilot study and randomized controlled trial of the mindful self-compassion program. *Journal of Clinical Psychology, 69*(1), 28–44.

Noone, S. J., & Hastings, R. (2010). Using acceptance and mindfulness-based workshops with support staff caring for adults with intellectual disabilities. *Mindfulness, 1*(2), 67–73.

Salzberg, S., & Goldstein, J. (2001). *Insight meditation*. Boulder: Sounds True.

Scottish Intercollegiate Guidelines Network (SIGN). (2010). *Non-pharmaceutical management of depression in adults*. Edinburgh: SIGN.

Segal, Z. V., Williams, J. M. G., & Teasdale, J. D. (2002). *Mindfulness-based cognitive therapy for depression: A new approach to preventing relapse*. New York: The Guilford Press.

Segal, Z. V., Williams, J. M. G., & Teasdale, J. D. (2013). *Mindfulness-based cognitive therapy for depression* (2nd ed.). New York: The Guilford Press.

Shapiro, S. L., Carlson, L. E., Astin, J. A., & Freedman, B. (2006). Mechanisms of mindfulness. *Journal of Clinical Psychology, 62*(3), 373–386.

Siegel, D. J. (2007). *The mindful brain: Reflection and attunement in the cultivation of well-being* (1st ed.). New York: W.W. Norton.

Singh, N. N., Lancioni, G. E., Winton, A. S., Curtis, W. J., Wahler, R. G., Sabaawi, M., et al. (2006). Mindful staff increase learning and reduce aggression in adults with developmental disabilities. *Research in Developmental Disabilities, 27*, 545–558.

Singh, N. N., Lancioni, G. E., Winto, A. S. W., Adkins, A. D., Singh, J., & Singh, A. N. (2007). Mindfulness training assists individuals with moderate mental retardation to maintain their community placements. *Behaviour Modification, 31*(6), 800–814.

Singh, N. N., Lancioni, G. E., Manikam, R., Winton, A. S. W., Singh, A. N. A., Singh, J., & Singh, A. D. A. (2011). A mindfulness-based strategy for self-management of aggressive behaviour in adolescents with autism. *Research in Autism Spectrum Disorders, 5*, 1153–1158.

Singh, N. N., Lancioni, G. E., & Karazsia, B. T. (2015). Effects of training staff in MBPBS on the use of physical restraints, staff stress and turnover, staff and peer injuries, and cost effectiveness in developmental disabilities. *Mindfulness, 6)*, 926.

Tang, Y. Y., Ma, Y., Wang, J., Fan, Y., Feng, S., Lu, Q., et al. (2007). Short-term meditation training improves attention and self-regulation. *Proceedings of the National Academy of Sciences of the United States of America, 104*(43), 17152–17156.

Teasdale, J. D., Moore, R. G., Hayhurst, H., Pope, M., Williams, S., & Segal, Z. V. (2002). Metacognitive awareness and prevention of relapse in depression: Empirical evidence. *Journal of Consulting and Clinical Psychology, 70,* 275–287.

Teper, R., & Inzlicht, M. (2013). Meditation, mindfulness and executive control: The importance of emotional acceptance and brain-based performance monitoring. *Social Cognitive Affective Neuroscience, 8,* 85–92.

Wells, A. (2007). Cognition about cognition: Metacognitive therapy and change in generalized anxiety disorder and social phobia. *Cognitive and Behavioral Practice, 14,* 18–25.

Williams, J., Crane, C., & Barnhofer, T. (2014). Mindfulness-based cognitive therapy for preventing relapse in recurrent depression: A randomized dismantling trial. *Journal of Consulting Clinical Psychology, 82,* 275–286.

Zellner Keller, B., Singh, N. N., & Winton, A. S. W. (2014). Mindfulness-based cognitive approach for seniors (MBCAS): Program development and implementation. *Mindfulness, 5*(4), 453–459.

10

Working with Others

In previous chapters we have already raised the topic of how best to involve other people in the therapeutic process and how to motivate them to support clients to access and benefit from CBT, complete 'homework' and implement coping and preventative strategies in their day-to-day lives.

The influence of the people who make up clients' immediate family, social and support networks is much more powerful and lasting than ours, as therapists, in determining psychological well-being. This is because they share a past history, spend more time and have strong and sometimes intimate relationships with our clients. They will also be there when therapy has long since ceased, having not just an immediate but also a long-lasting influence on our clients' lives. Compared to the few hour-long sessions that a CBT therapist can spend with a client, their family, friends and staff have a wealth of time and extensive experience on which to base their knowledge of the client and the client's behaviour and psychological make-up.

This does not mean that a therapist cannot make valuable contributions to the formulation and the amelioration of the client's psychological distress. Often the views of an interested and qualified outsider can throw new and helpful light on what has become an insurmountable problem for a closely knit group of people. It *does* mean that when we work with people who themselves may not be able to fully comprehend, remember and report on past events and their own internal states, we are wise to respect the knowledge and insights of others and to take advantage of what can often be a wealth of vital information to aid us in our psychological understanding.

This chapter will describe the roles and influence we think other people can have when we work as CBT therapists with adults with intellectual disabilities. We include in 'other people' immediate family members, support staff and health and social services professionals.

We will not dwell on role of the 'general public' although we recognise that cultural and social attitudes and behaviours towards people with intellectual disabilities have a significant impact on their well-being. There is a substantial literature (see Scior 2011 for a review) on this topic and it is generally found that attitudes towards people with intellectual disabilities are more negative than towards people with physical and sensory disabilities, although not as negative as towards people with mental health problems. For example, when people were asked by the Office for Disability Issues (2009) whether they would feel comfortable if someone with a disability moved next door to them, 76% said 'yes' when it concerned someone with a physical or sensory disability, 49% if it was a person with an intellectual disability and only 27% felt comfortable with someone with a mental health problem as a neighbour. If we are to tackle the impact on psychological well-being that such predominantly negative attitudes are likely to have on our clients, especially those with an intellectual disability *and* mental health problems, we should consider the initiatives that are based on Community Psychology principles (e.g. Orford 2008), where the focus is on empowerment of marginalised groups of people, including people with intellectual disabilities and mental health problems. Community psychologists try to bring about (by means of a system-based approach) social change to address mental health and well-being because they recognise that people's social settings and the systems with which they interact affect (and often cause) their psychological problems and are influential in shaping the solutions they devise to cope, and how effective these coping strategies turn out to be. For community psychologists, disempowered groups are helped not just by therapies and interventions that only involve the individual members of those groups, but by working with and strengthening their communities.

For example, when a person with intellectual disabilities is too frightened to go out and travel by bus because she has experienced taunting and bullying from school children, the community psychologist may contact the local school and provide advice and interventions (e.g. drama workshops where pupils meet people with intellectual disabilities and work with them) to change attitudes of pupils towards people with disabilities, to tolerate difference and to develop a deeper awareness of the adverse impact of bullying on people who are already marginalised. In this way, the external cause of the psychological distress is addressed. That is, we try to reduce the incidence of bullying of adults with intellectual disabilities in public spaces rather than just providing the client with 'coping strategies' to deal with her anxiety symptoms when she leaves her house or thinks about going out. We fully endorse the community psychology approach and its theoretical underpinnings and have used it exclusively or side by side individual therapeutic approaches such as CBT.

The 'others' discussed in this chapter are more closely related to our clients and their lives are interwoven, either through family or friendship ties or through their professional roles and responsibilities.

Family Members

Four out of five people with intellectual disabilities are supported by their families, and family care is the predominant care provided until well into middle age (Jacques 2003). When adults with intellectual disabilities living in the family home attend CBT sessions, they are likely to be accompanied by one or both of their parents although in later life siblings may have taken over the general care, including supporting and accompanying the client to come to therapy.

There is a traditional view (and a substantial research literature to support it) that having a child with intellectual disabilities has nothing but negative effects on the parents and the family as a whole. This view is now challenged and many family members report that there are also positive effects and rewards. Services are no longer designed to respond to the family's 'pathological reaction' to the birth of a child with intellectual disabilities but now aim to support and augment the assumed adaptive functioning of family care.

> Stainton and Besser's (1998) research indicates that the positives of having a child or adult family member with intellectual disabilities include:
> The person with intellectual disabilities being a source of joy and happiness
> Having an increased sense of purpose and priorities
> Expanded personal and social networks
> Increased spirituality
> The person with intellectual disabilities being a source of family unity and closeness
> Developing increased tolerance and understanding, personal growth and strength
> The person with intellectual disabilities having a positive impact on others in the community.

But the challenges that caring for a close relative with intellectual disabilities pose for families should not be disregarded. Assuming that families can always easily cope and do not need responsive and family-centred support services would be naive and ill-informed. Research (Seltzer et al. 2012) involving older parents caring for their sons and daughters with intellectual disabilities found that these parents were significantly disadvantaged in terms of economic factors, physical and mental health, and social status when compared to their peers. It must be pointed out though that rather than attributing the cause of these distinct disadvantages solely to the presence and needs of the person with the intellectual disabilities, many relatives in Selzer's study report that unsympathetic and unhelpful interactions with professionals are often the main cause of stress and frustration. Family members are particularly concerned that professionals fail to communicate clearly and honestly, and do not appear to consider the family's opinions. Instead of acting as a supportive influence on the well-being of the family, social, educational and health professionals are often perceived as ineffectual at best and adding to the family's problems at worst. That many of the interventions on offer are reported to *add* to the difficulties of these families rather than reduce them should be a matter of concern for all of us working in intellectual disabilities services.

Mental health services for people with intellectual disabilities are by no means an exception in this respect and it is important that when we first meet a relative we anticipate and be sensitive to the possibly negative expectations that family members may have of us due to their previous experiences of health and other services. During the assessment phase we can negotiate with the client how the voice of the family member(s) can be heard without interfering with the therapeutic relationship. Subtle decisions have to be made about when it is helpful and when it may be counterproductive to involve parents or other family members in therapy sessions.

There are many ways in which we can ensure that family members are not made to feel they are being excluded or patronised whilst at the same time respecting the client's right to confidentiality. If a co-therapist is available, you can see your client while your colleague conducts a parallel session with the family. You can then choose to all come together at the end of the session to exchange information and perhaps agree on action plans. It may, on the other hand, be more appropriate to ask the family member to join some of the sessions or parts of these sessions (usually the end part) so that the therapist and the client can explain the work that has been done so far and/or the psychological formulation that they have developed together. If the client is comfortable with sharing information, it can help family members to feel part of the therapeutic process and gain a better understanding of the psychological principles that are the foundation for the coping skills that are being recommended. It is our experience that understanding and feeling included in the therapy increases the motivation of the parent or sibling to support their relative with intellectual disabilities in completing 'homework', diary keeping, implementing new skills and maintaining established coping strategies.

There are occasions when on first meeting, the therapist is overwhelmed by the relatives' psychological needs and sometimes by their apparent unwillingness or inability to listen and have a reciprocal conversation. The way they present may well be the end product of years of battling with various services in order to get the best for their son or daughter and an anxiety about not being listened to and not being taken seriously.

We have met parents who report that they have struggled to understand what professionals consider to be appropriate services for their adult sons and daughters because underlying service principles such as *independence, social role valorisation* and *individual choice* are foreign (and often badly explained) concepts and do not easily fit in with their culture and values and what they perceive to be their roles and responsibilities as parents. Parents often consider these responsibilities to be the same as those relevant to parents of young children and they may struggle to see why issues such as independence, valued adult roles, confidentiality, choice and age-appropriate activities are raised.

A particular sensitive subject that is a frequent worry for parents is the freedom that usually comes with adulthood to express one's sexuality and to seek out sexual partners. Most service providers would support these rights for adults with intellectual disabilities in principle and may take active steps to ensure that they are respected (e.g. by providing their clients with sex education, contraceptive advice and opportunities for them to meet and spend private time with a potential sexual partner). But they may not inform clients' family members, as they would consider this to be a breach of confidentiality. Parents may not have the same attitude to their son's or daughter's sexual freedom and may be primarily concerned with their safety and the real possibility of sexual abuse and exploitation. They may view adults with intellectual disabilities as 'eternal children' for whom sexual activity is wholly inappropriate. Health and social professionals, on the other hand, may consider this to be an unacceptable authoritarian stance and for this reason may provide the client with services and support unbeknownst to the parents.

As therapists, it is not always possible to address the differences that exist in attitudes and aims of parents and service providers and the resultant hostility and suspicion between parties. However, because CBT has amongst its core concepts the power of *underlying assumptions* influencing thoughts, feelings and behaviour it is important for us to consider the family's values, aims and expectations in respect to the person with intellectual disabilities as they cannot fail to affect the client's cognitive mediating events and the opportunities they have to achieve their therapeutic goals.

In order to work with family members in a constructive manner it can sometimes be useful to introduce Narrative Therapy methods (White and Epston 1990), which can be done using *metacompetent adherence* (Whittington and Grey 2014; see Chap. 2), without corrupting the CBT model. For example, 'externalising' is a concept that was introduced to the field of family therapy in the early 1980s and is best summed up in the phrase 'the person is not the problem, the problem is the problem'. We meet clients and their families who think of psychological problems as 'internal' to us, as if they represent something about the 'inner self'. Narrative therapists see problems as socially constructed and created over time and use every opportunity to show their clients that they and their problems are not one and the same. One way of doing this is by asking questions in which the adjectives that people use to describe themselves or others ('I am a depressed person'; 'My son is a depressive') are changed into nouns ('How long has this depression been around?'). Another way to externalise the problem involves asking questions in a way that invites people to personify problems. For instance, when working with a young woman who often found herself embroiled in verbal confrontations, we asked her to name the verbal aggression as a separate entity (she chose the name 'Mrs Shouty') and an externalising question might be, 'How does Mrs Shouty get you into trouble?' or 'When does Mrs Shouty bother you most?'

Drane and Coles (2015) describe how a young woman with chronic low mood externalised her problem of getting out of bed in the morning to go to work as the 'Bed Lover' and the force that could help her overcome her depressive symptoms as 'Elephant Bed'. She was able to describe and draw how Elephant Bed could defeat Bed Lover by stamping on and squirting water at him. Externalising both her problems and her ability to overcome her problems helped her to open up and discuss her negative emotions with the therapist and with her mother.

By externalising the problem, space is created between the client and the problem and this enables the client to begin to revise their relationship with the problem. It also helps family members to recognise their role in aggravating or reducing the problem and challenges their assumption that CBT should 'sort out' the client. Externalising is linked to a particular tradition of thought often referred to as post-structuralism (e.g. Thomas 2002), which places an emphasis on the use of language, questions of power and the ways in which meaning and identities are constructed. Externalising the problem with clients and their families can be very useful when agreeing on therapeutic goals and reviewing progress. It avoids a blaming game, can help people think about power dynamics afresh and can make them more aware of the language they use and how such language influences the way they think about problems. It also allows them to consider their own and others' perceived roles in their family and wider social networks, all of which are compatible with CBT principles and desired outcomes.

But sometimes, even after using narrative methods, the needs, perspectives and opinions of the various family members may continue to differ radically from those of the client and it may be necessary to address these differences by negotiation. There may also be occasions when strict confidentiality (not sharing information with the family) is more appropriate than entering into discussions with the family to attempt to build bridges and reach agreements. For example, whereas it may be an effective and constructive strategy to negotiate a young adult's bedtime with his deeply religious parents and in the process address his need for independence and choice on the one hand and developing a sense of responsibility and self-care on the other, discussing his aim to meet a same-sex partner in a private and safe environment may not be. Instead, as therapists we might in some instances liaise with social workers and other colleagues to consider alternative housing options and other ways in which the client can express his sexuality without causing rifts and distress within the family.

We also meet many adults with intellectual disabilities who present with complex psychological problems where family members are likely to have been the main cause of their difficulties. This may be because the client has been abused or neglected by some or all members of their family, other family members' mental health needs may have adversely affected them, or parents' divorce may have caused them distress. In many such cases it is not safe or viable to involve certain family members and the focus of the therapy should then be on the client's ability and the opportunities open to them to develop new and supportive social networks to compensate for the loss of past family relationships.

Support Staff

Although a large number of adults with intellectual disabilities remain in their family home or with close family members throughout their lives, others will reside in accommodation, either shared or alone, supported by staff from statutory services or independent organisations. So another important modification in the use of CBT when working with adults with intellectual disabilities is to take account of and consider the role of support workers in the process of therapy. As with family members, CBT therapists may decide that the client is best seen alone and that they will benefit most from therapy if all that is discussed is kept strictly confidential. But in many cases the input of a support worker can be very useful. For example, during the assessment phase a support worker can provide the therapist with demographic details and describe recent relevant events if the client is unable or reticent to do so. They may be a reassuring presence for the client especially during the first few sessions and may motivate clients to continue attendance to therapy sessions and also support them in practical ways that make consistent attendance more likely, such as time keeping and providing transport. As mentioned earlier in this chapter, support workers can also throw light on the causes and maintenance factors of clients' psychological problems and may have detailed knowledge of past events.

Explaining the formulation to a support worker (with the client's consent) can ensure the client is enabled to use their coping strategies and maintain their improved psychological health long after the therapy sessions have ended. The involvement of support workers can also increase the chances that a timely re-referral is made if clients experience deterioration in their condition.

In practice, we find that some support workers are keen and very able to take on these roles whereas others show no interest and may even actively discourage the client from attending therapy and tackling their problems.

> A typical job description for a community or residential support worker post reads like this:
>
> - Provide practical and emotional support and assist people to undertake a range of social, recreational and developmental activities as mature adults in the local community, promoting lifelong learning.
> - Advise in an advocacy role as well as promoting the concept of self-advocacy.
> - Build and maintain close working relationships with family, friends and relevant agencies, dealing with all information on a confidential basis.
> - Assist individuals with the day-to-day domestic management of their home and related budgeting, to include personal budgeting.
> - Contribute to the preparation and implementation of Person Centred Planning, identifying agreed objectives, assisting in the production of relevant reports and participating in appropriate developmental activities that ultimately lead to the achievement of identified goals.

Such job descriptions cover a wide range of roles and responsibilities and the workload is invariably high and time pressured. But mention of 'emotional support' and 'close working relationships with relevant agencies' and 'participating in appropriate developmental activities' suggests that, according to their employment contract, support workers not only can but should be involved in psychological interventions, in the same way as that they are expected to be involved in supporting the client in domestic and social activities.

The involvement of a support worker can make the therapeutic process accessible for the client and increase the chance that they will benefit from therapy. Support workers can be especially helpful when it comes to the completion of homework tasks and to implementing coping strategies in their day-to-day lives. Rose et al. (2005) found that having a support worker accompany the client to CBT anger management group sessions resulted in better and longer lasting outcomes, suggesting that the support workers were able to assist participants in practising their anger management skills outside the session. We found that staff members who facilitated anger management groups were able to prompt their clients outside the therapy sessions to apply their coping skills (Rose et al. 2015). Positive outcomes included service users appearing calmer and more comfortable with discussing their feelings, not only in the group setting but also outside of the group, resulting in better relationships between service users and staff members.

Managers of the day services where the groups were held, who were interviewed by Rose and colleagues, mentioned that the strategies learned in the group could be prompted by staff and so were more likely to be applied by service users in 'real life':

> You could actually see evidence of them (service users) trying to put in place what they've learned and experienced in the group.

We have found (Willner et al. 2013) that training support staff to deliver therapeutic group interventions in their work setting as 'lay therapists' has many potential advantages. Firstly, members of staff become familiar with the coping techniques that participants learn about in the therapy sessions and so are in a good position to provide their clients with ongoing support to apply these skills outside of the sessions. They are also able to share knowledge and skills of therapeutic methods with other staff members in the service and to share information about service users' progress. A further consideration relates to the current economic and political climate in which the squeeze on mental health services has given rise to a need to think pragmatically about how psychological skills can be made more widely available. As support staff typically spend a substantial proportion of their time with service users over the course of a working week and an important part of their role is to provide direct support for people with mental health problems, they present as an obvious choice to train to deliver psychological interventions. However, we recommend that such psychological support is only provided for types of psychological problems that are suitable for 'low-intensity' CBT interventions (Bennett-Levy et al. 2010) and with the assurance that robust supervision arrangements for the support workers are in place. Clients who present with more serious and complex symptoms will require the input of a more highly qualified therapist.

In cases where the presenting problems are more complex and a qualified CBT therapist needs to conduct the therapy, support workers can still play a valuable and prominent role. We have found, though, that including a support worker in sessions and motivating them to support their client in their quest to improve psychological well-being can be a complex task, particularly when the client is perceived to be 'challenging' and the client/support worker relationship is fragile. Hassiotis et al. (2012) note in their therapist manual that the involvement of the support worker must be carefully managed so that the client doesn't become too dependent and rely too heavily on the support worker during the course of treatment as one of the fundamental aims of CBT is to empower individuals to become 'their own therapist'. If a client relies too heavily on the presence and prompts of the support worker, he or she may not integrate CBT techniques as coping mechanisms when that member of staff is absent.

Co-working with support staff will invariably raise important issues relating to confidentiality. Confidentiality ensures that information disclosed to the therapist is not shared unless agreed by the client beforehand. It is an important part of the therapeutic process that allows trust to be built up between the client and the therapist. The therapist, therefore, needs to establish how much and what information the client is willing to disclose to the support worker. Lasky and Riva (2006) found that in a therapy group setting, successful treatment depends on individuals feeling safe enough to disclose personal information. The therapist, whether in a group or individual therapy setting, needs to determine during the assessment phase what the client is willing to share with members of staff, and then must make sure that the support workers who attend the sessions will respect confidentiality.

We (Stenfert Kroese et al. 2016) found that when we asked people to tell us about their experiences of a trauma-focused CBT group, most people found the presence of their own support worker reassuring. For example:

> I was really glad I went with a support worker, because if it got difficult they knew you and could say go out for five minutes and leave the room. I find it difficult to ask or say with new people in the group.

Like Lasky and Riva (2006) we found that our group members valued safety and trust. As they all had experienced severely traumatising events in their past, their evaluation of the group was often phrased in terms of how safe they felt in that setting, for example:

Knowing you could go talking to people you could trust.

Although it makes individual as well as group therapy more accessible to clients with complex problems, there are potential disadvantages to inviting clients to bring a support worker with them to therapy sessions. As we have described in Chap. 8, it can affect continuity, as often different support staff accompany the service user to the sessions. Also, we have found that some support staff may at times act in an inappropriate and sometimes disrespectful manner towards the clients. As therapists we continue to invite support staff as otherwise a significant number of service users could not benefit from our CBT interventions. But where group therapy is concerned, we now ask support staff to attend a training session so that they are aware of the ethical and psychological principles on which the intervention is based, and their managers will be asked to allocate the same support worker throughout the course of the group intervention to avoid undue disruption to the group dynamics. We provide staff with a leaflet that outlines the main purpose and principles of therapy, whether it be individual or group therapy, and a number of 'ground rules' for them to adhere to:

- Encourage clients to share their experiences and to participate fully
- Be supportive of honest disclosures, don't judge or make fun of them
- Empower clients to talk rather than talking for them
- Maintain confidentiality at all times
- Help clients to understand the learning points of the session and the instructions for exercises
- Reinforce learning outside of therapy by helping clients with completing diaries and other work outside of the session, and answer any questions raised by your client.

(Adapted from Rose, *Information for people supporting group members leaflet*, personal communication)

We have found (Stenfert Kroese et al. 2014) that support staff are likely to expect very little good to come from CBT work and may lack enthusiasm for supporting their clients to attend the sessions. How can we as therapists help to avoid such negative attitudes from developing? One psychological concept that is helpful in this context is that of reciprocity. Reciprocity refers to the balance between how much a person invests in a relationship on the one hand and how much they feel they get from that relationship. In a work setting, if employees perceive that their investment in the relationships they develop with clients and other workers far outweighs the positive outcomes for them, they are likely to eventually develop emotional exhaustion and burn out (van Horn et al. 2001).

If we want to engage support workers in the therapeutic process we need to assess what we can provide them with that they may value and what they may be able to get out of their 'investment' in the relationships with their clients and with us and spending time and effort with the client to help them put their CBT coping skills into practice. What outcomes are perceived as positive will of course vary. In our experience, being treated as a valued colleague and being consulted and informed throughout the therapy process is much appreciated by most (but not all) support workers. Findings from one of our studies (Stenfert Kroese et al. 2014), where we interviewed 11 staff, indicate that support workers may perceive themselves as peripheral to the CBT and as only having a practical support role (e.g. 'to get him there and back') or that they should not be involved at all: 'This is nothing to do with me, my role is quite different.'

A significant number of support staff may not consider the CBT approach to have any new, additional qualities over and above what they themselves do in order to address clients' psychological distress (e.g. 'It's repeating what I've been saying'). We also found that they had little or no knowledge of the CBT approach, for example, 'What's cognitive? I haven't a clue.' Most of the staff we interviewed indicated that for them the desired outcomes of the CBT intervention concerned other people's convenience or welfare, such as 'I hope [name of therapist] can talk some sense into him', 'for [name of client] to stop lying' and that they would like clients to accept responsibility for their own actions, to get on better with other people and not to commit suicide. The psychological and general well-being of the client was rarely mentioned. This tendency may be because most training that staff receive encourages them to think in behavioural terms (challenging versus adaptive behaviours) rather than considering their clients' emotional problems and well-being.

It is therefore important to provide support staff with information about the principles and purpose of CBT, not just to explain how they may play a role in the therapeutic process but also to build a reciprocal relationship with them so that they are more likely to become (and remain) motivated and engaged in the work they do with the client.

The research that explored the experiences of 'lay therapists' during the Willner randomised control trial (RCT) (Stimpson et al. 2013) also indicates that the training, supervision and increased responsibilities that go with the new role can provide support staff with a welcome opportunity to expand and diversify their knowledge and skills, enable them to contribute to service development, and support service users more effectively. The lay therapists described their involvement in the CBT groups as an enjoyable, rewarding and productive experience. They identified a range of skills that they had learned and considered important, including being able to forge collaborative relationships with clients. The concept of collaboration between the lay therapists and group members through exchange of ideas and working together captures the essence of the therapeutic relationship in CBT (Gilbert and Leahy 2007) and suggests a perceived reciprocity, predicting job satisfaction and reduced risk of work-related stress and eventual burnout amongst staff.

We firmly believe that providing support staff with good training and supervision can prevent the deterioration in morale and standards, such as witnessed to such an extreme degree in the privately run Winterbourne View Hospital. The investigation into this scandal (Department of Health, Final Report 2012) revealed amongst other causative factors a lack of training and supervision which, in a closed and controlling environment, produced a toxic and bullying culture where some staff, instead of caring and supporting the clients with intellectual disabilities, became extremely callous and abusive.

When we asked clients with mental health problems and intellectual disabilities as well as their support and professional staff (Stenfert Kroese et al. 2013) what they thought would make a good worker, clients considered it important that staff members receive training:

> People should have the right training for the job so they can do their job properly. People don't always know what the job involves.

They also mentioned that communication is an important area to provide training in. One client noted that having students from the various professions on placement was a positive thing for everyone, perhaps noticing that having a 'learner' observing clinical practice inspired everyone to be on their best behaviour.

Good clinical supervision separated from the management hierarchy was stressed by many of the staff members who participated in this study.

Training methods preferred by staff, other than standard classroom teaching, included:

- mentoring schemes
- peer supervision
- having a clinical lead post alongside the manager
- reciprocal secondment/shadowing schemes with colleagues in mental health services
- a clinical information group on mental health
- joint work with mental health colleagues

A number of staff did not feel comfortable receiving clinical supervision from their manager and preferred to receive supervision from an experienced clinician not in a managerial position to them.

Many support workers were disappointed with the training opportunities available in their organisation. A number of staff reported that they were to a large extent self-educated in mental health issues. They were keen that training happened in the workplace and as an ongoing process, with 'refresher' courses available on a regular basis.

The community team professionals who took part in this research also stressed the importance of including support staff who work in residential settings in training initiatives as they consider them to be highly influential in determining the psychological well-being of clients:

> Where someone [with mental health problems] is living in a care home, they are reliant on those people who care for them and so if they're not caring for them properly, they need education

and

> because I think some of the lower paid workers actually get the brunt of some of the hard parts of the work and they might be faced with something that's really difficult and identifying that at an early stage.

Health and Social Services Professionals

We sometimes find ourselves liaising with other professionals involved in our clients' general health and social care. We know from a number of studies (e.g. Gill et al. 2002) that most health and social services staff do not receive much, if any, training in how to adjust their practice for people with intellectual disabilities. This very often results in the person with intellectual disabilities receiving a service that is below par or receiving no service at all.

The lack of good physical health, both in primary and in secondary care, has come under much scrutiny in the last decade. Mencap's reports *Treat Me Right!* (2004) and *Death by Indifference* (2007) and the Disability Rights Commission's *Equal Treatment: Closing the Gap* (2006) highlight poorer health outcomes for people with intellectual disabilities, poor communication between professionals and people with intellectual disabilities, a lack of understanding of their health needs, a lack of user-friendly literature to support informed choices, poor training for professionals, poor access to primary care, a lack of health screening and poor treatment in general practice. The Sir Jonathan Michael's enquiry *Healthcare for All* (2008) called for radical changes, finding that people with intellectual disabilities have poorer health, have higher levels of unmet need, experience unequal treatment and a lack of 'reasonable adjustments' being made for them.

In particular, general practitioners (GPs) who in the UK are the central coordinators of health care are sometimes at a loss regarding what to do for their patients with intellectual disabilities and although their attitudes to this client group is generally positive, they were often unwilling to adapt their behaviour and practice (e.g. longer sessions) to accommodate them (Gill et al. 2002). When people with mental health problems and intellectual disabilities present themselves (or are referred by others), GPs may resort to focusing on the problems experienced by the carers and support workers, rather than the well-being of the patient with the intellectual disabilities and so will often prescribe psychotropic medication to reduce the patient's 'challenging behaviours'. A recent report (Sheenan et al. 2015) refers to this tendency as the 'chemical cosh' which has resulted in a large proportion of people with intellectual disabilities being given powerful antipsychotics commonly used for people with a diagnosis of severe mental illness such as schizophrenia or bipolar disorder in order to control behaviour deemed problematic by carers. In this study over two-thirds of the 9000+ GP patients with learning disabilities treated with powerful antipsychotic drugs did not have a record or diagnosis of severe mental illness. The authors describe this as concerning; it is difficult to justify the use of these strong drugs because they can have problematic side effects such as sedation, weight gain and metabolic changes that can lead to diabetes, restlessness, stiffness and tremors (tardive dyskinesia). These symptoms can affect health and quality of life and, most pertinent of all for people with intellectual disabilities, cognitive and executive functioning.

As CBT therapists we have worked with people who, after presenting as attentive and engaged, turn up for their session the following week with a 'glazed' look and unable to engage with us in any meaningful way or benefit from talking therapy because they have been prescribed psychotropic medication or have been given PRN. Moncrieff et al. (2013) after interviewing people who had taken neuroleptic drugs conclude that they 'produce a state that is characterised by sedation, lethargy, flattening of emotional responses, indifference and feelings of impaired mental functioning' (p. 226). Houghton (2016) suggests that, although we must acknowledge the limitations of our knowledge of medication and how it should be prescribed, as responsible clinicians we must take every opportunity to 'gently enquire and explore issues around medication with colleagues in a respectful and curious way' (p. 12).

We must make sure when we start a course of CBT that other professionals are aware of the importance of continuity and stability during therapy and that for a set period of time other interventions are, whenever possible, coordinated and not contraindicative for our planned CBT work. This goes for health as well as social interventions. For people to be able to meaningfully engage with any talking therapy, they require to be reasonably healthy, safe and stable (Herman 1997) in order to benefit.

Specialist Services

Most parts of the UK now have locality-based community multidisciplinary teams (CTs) to promote general and mental health and well-being for adults with intellectual disabilities, as well as community inclusion (National LD Professional Senate 2015). They are made up of a number of health and social service professionals usually including social workers, specialist psychiatrists, community nurses, psychologists, speech and language therapists and occupational therapists. All these professionals can play an important role in the lives of our clients, and it can at times be vital to the outcome of our therapy that we liaise and share information with them. For example, when during the course of our work we discover that a client lives in an unsuitable, deprived or even abusive environment, it is our duty to alert and work with social workers to address these problems and service deficiencies.

Psychiatrists and community nurses may already be involved with clients who have serious mental health problems and can be important informants and allies in improving the mental well-being of the client. Speech and language therapists are experts in communication, and we have found it helpful to consult them when in doubt about how to best interact with clients who may have limited verbal comprehension and/or expression or a speech impediment that makes them difficult to understand. Occupational therapists are not only experts in adaptive functioning related to home, work and community environments but also have useful skills in relaxation and sensory integration. The specialist knowledge and experience that these colleagues in specialist intellectual disabilities services have can greatly benefit us as CBT therapists and can complement the interventions that we can offer our clients.

There may at times be some potential for conflicting views due to various professions having different explanatory frames of reference and different approaches to psychological problems. For example, psychiatrists and psychologists differ in the way they view the origins, maintenance and treatment of mental health problems. The BPS-DCP's position statement (ref) raises concerns over the use of classification systems such as the *Diagnostic and Statistical Manual of Mental Disorders* (DSM 5) and the *International Classification of Diseases: Classification of Mental and Behavioural Disorders* (ICD-10). We agree that these systems are limited in their capacity to provide a clear understanding of complex mental health problems, and we are concerned about the scientific basis of the American Psychiatry Association's *Diagnostic and Statistical Manual of Mental Disorders* (DSM) because it is more categorical than diagnostic, with validity and reliability of the system questioned. Yet diagnostic classifications are commonly used in a range of clinical and commercial fields—psychiatry, health insurance and the pharmaceutical industry. The DCP position statement stresses that a formulation approach is preferable to a diagnostic model as:

> there is a large and growing body of evidence suggesting that the experiences described in diagnostic terms may be better understood as a response to psychosocial factors such as loss, trauma, poverty, inequality, unemployment, discrimination, and other social, relational and societal factors … we need to move towards a system which is no longer based on a 'disease' model.

As CBT therapists we subscribe to the formulation approach. However, we also consider the role of our psychiatrist and nursing colleagues important in the care of our clients and do not consider our different theoretical stances necessarily an obstacle to good and complementary multidisciplinary working. We consider a good community team to have the capacity for effective dialogue with effective processes for decision-making and the ability to engage in constructive conflict. Lucy Johnstone (2014) has written about how to make such dialogue most effective and makes an excellent case for the introduction of team-based formulation, where as a group (whether as a reflective-practice group or as a drop-in discussion forum), the multidisciplinary team discusses and plans their interventions to meet their clients' needs, using the same framework and information gathering process as individual therapists when, in collaboration with their client, they develop testable formulations and then base their treatment choices on these formulations.

Key Points
- When working with people with ID, there may be a number of other people who we may need to be in contact with, not just to gather background information but also to recruit them as allies who can play an influential and long-term role in implementing and maintaining psychological and environmental change.
- We need to carefully consider when it is and when it is not suitable to involve other people so that we respect the client's right to confidentiality.
- Staff report that they receive very little training in mental health and psychological issues and sometimes we may need to spend time with caregivers and staff to make sure that they understand and agree with the CBT model and the formulation.
- As therapists we must liaise with our health and social services colleagues and ensure that the various interventions received by clients are well coordinated and are not detrimental to each other.
- Family carers and support workers as well as health and social services professionals can complement the CBT approach and improve the chances of significant and enduring improvements in psychological well-being.

References

Bennett-Levy, J., Richards, D., Farrand, P., Christensen, H., Griffiths, K., Kavanagh, D., Klein, B., Lau, M. A., Proudfoot, J., Ritterband, L., White, J., & Williams, C. (2010). *Oxford guide to low intensity CBT interventions*. Oxford: Oxford University Press.

Department of Health. (2012). Transforming care: A national response to Winterbourne View Hospital. Final report. https://www.gov.uk/government/uploads/system/uploads/attachment_data/file/213215/final-report.pdf

Disability Rights Commission. (2006). *Equal treatment: Closing the gap. A formal investigation into physical health inequalities experienced by people with learning disabilities and/or mental health problems*. London: Disability Rights Commission.

Division of Clinical Psychology. (2014). Position statement on the classification of behaviour and experience in relation to functional psychiatric diagnoses time for a paradigm shift. http://www.bps.org.uk/system/files/Public%20files/cat-1325.pdf

Drane, E., & Coles, S. (2015). Goodbye, bed lover: Reconceptualising depression – A narrative approach. *The Bulletin of the Faculty for People with Intellectual Disabilities, 13*(2), 15–21.

Gilbert, P., & Leahy, R. L. (2007). *The therapeutic relationship in cognitive behavioural psychotherapies*. London: Routledge.

Gill, F., Stenfert Kroese, B., & Rose, J. (2002). General practitioners' attitudes to patients who have learning disabilities. *Psychological Medicine, 32*(8), 1445–1455.

Hassiotis, A., Serfaty, M., Azam, K., Martin, S., Strydom, A., & King, M. (2012). *A manual of cognitive behaviour therapy for people with mild learning disabilities and common mental disorders: A training guide to help professional therapists in treating people with communication and cognitive problems*. Camden & Islington NHS Foundation Trust/University College London. https://www.ucl.ac.uk/ciddr/resources

Herman, J. L. (1997). *Trauma and recovery*. New York: Basic Books.

Houghton, P. (2016). Joining the debate around psychiatric medication. *Clinical Psychology Forum, 286*, 10–14.

Jacques, R. (2003). Family issues. *Psychiatry, 2*(9), 39–42.

Johnstone, L. (2014). Using formulation in teams. In L. Johnstone & R. Dallos (Eds.), *Formulation in psychology and psychotherapy: Making sense of people's problems* (2nd ed.). Hove: Routledge.

Lasky, G. B., & Riva, M. T. (2006). Confidentiality and privileged communication in group psychotherapy. *International Journal of Group Psychotherapy, 56*(4), 455–476.
MENCAP. (2004). *Treat me right!* London: MENCAP.
MENCAP. (2007). *Death by indifference.* London: MENCAP.
Michael, J., & Richardson, A. (2008). Healthcare for all: The independent enquiry into access to healthcare for people with learning disabilities. *Tizard Learning Disability Review, 13*(4), 28–34.
Moncrieff, J., Cohen, D., & Mason, J. (2013). The patient's dilemma: An analysis of users' experiences of taking neuroleptic drugs. In S. Coles, S. Keenan, & B. Diamond (Eds.), *Madness contested: Power and practice.* Ross-on-Wye: PCCS Books.
National LD Professional Senate. (2015). *Delivering effective specialist community learning disabilities health team support to people with learning disabilities and their families or carers.* A briefing paper on service specifications and best practice for professionals, NHS commissioners, CQC and providers of community learning disabilities health team. https://www.bps.org.uk/.../national_ld_professional_senate_guidelines_for_cldt_speci
Orford, J. (2008). *Community psychology: Challenges, controversies and emerging consensus.* London: Wiley.
Rose, J., Loftus, M., Flint, B., & Carey, L. (2005). Factors associated with the efficacy of a group intervention for anger in people with intellectual disabilities. *British Journal of Clinical Psychology, 44*(3), 305–317.
Rose, N., Rose, J., Stenfert Kroese, B., Stimpson, A., MacMahon, P., Jahoda, A., Townson, J., Felce, D., Hood, K., & Willner, P. (2015). Managers' views of the effects on their service of hosting a cognitive-behavioural anger management group. *Advances in Mental health and Intellectual Disabilities, 9*(1), 19–29.
Scior, K. (2011). Public awareness, attitudes and beliefs regarding intellectual disability: A systematic review. *Research in Developmental Disabilities, 32*(6), 2164–2182.
Seltzer, M. M., Floyd, F. J., Song, J., Greenberg, J. S., & Hong, J. (2012). Midlife and aging parents of adults with intellectual and developmental disabilities: Impacts of lifelong parenting. *American Journal of Intellectual and Developmental Disabilities, 116*(6), 479–499.
Sheenan, R., Hassiotis, A., Walters, K., Osborn, D., Strydom, A., & Horsfall, L. (2015). Mental illness, challenging behaviour, and psychotropic drug prescribing in people with intellectual disability: UK population based cohort study. *British Medical Journal, 351.* doi:10.1136/bmj.h4326

Stainton, T., & Besser, H. (1998). The positive impact of children with an intellectual disability on the family. *Journal of Intellectual and Developmental Disabilities, 23*, 55–70.

Stenfert Kroese, B., Rose, J., Heer, K., & O'Brien, A. (2013). Mental health services for adults with intellectual disabilities – What do service users and staff think of them? *Journal of Applied Research in Intellectual Disabilities, 26*(1), 3–13.

Stenfert Kroese, B., Jahoda, A., Pert, C., Trower, P., Dagnan, D., & Selkirk, M. (2014). Staff expectations and views of cognitive behaviour therapy (CBT) for adults with intellectual disabilities. *Journal of Applied Research in Intellectual Disabilities, 27*(2), 145–153.

Stenfert Kroese, B., Willott, S., Taylor, F., Smith, P., Graham, R., Rutter, T., Stott, A., & Willner, P. (2016). Trauma-focussed cognitive-behaviour therapy for people with mild intellectual disabilities: Outcomes of a pilot study. *Advances in Mental Health and Intellectual Disabilities, 10*(5), 299–310.

Stimpson, A., Stenfert Kroese, B., MacMahon, P., Rose, N., Townson, J., Felce, D., Hood, K., Jahoda, A., Rose, J., & Willner, P. (2013). The experiences of staff taking on the role of lay therapist in a group-based cognitive behavioural therapy anger management intervention for people with intellectual disabilities. *Journal of Applied Research in Intellectual Disabilities, 26*(1), 63–70.

Thomas, L. (2002). Poststructuralism and therapy – What's it all about. *International Journal of Narrative Therapy and Community Work, 2002*(2), 85–89.

van Horn, J. E., Schaufeli, W. B., & Taris, T. W. (2001). Lack of reciprocity among Dutch teachers: Validation of reciprocity indices and their relation to stress and wellbeing. *Work and Stress, 15*, 191–213.

White, M., & Epston, D. (1990). *Narrative means to therapeutic ends.* New York: W.W. Norton.

Whittington, A., & Grey, N. (2014). *How to become a more effective CBT therapist – Mastering metacompetence in clinical practice.* Oxford: Wiley Blackwell.

Willner, P., Rose, J., Jahoda, A., Stenfert Kroese, B., Felce, D., Cohen, D., MacMahon, P., Stimpson, A., Rose, N., Gillespie, D., Shead, J., Lammie, C., Woodgate, C., Townson, J., Nuttall, J., & Hood, K. (2013). Group-based cognitive-behavioural anger management for people with mild to moderate intellectual disabilities: Cluster randomised controlled trial. *The British Journal of Psychiatry, 203*(4), 288–296.

11

Making a Real Difference

It would be good to able to say that since the publication of the first book on CBT and people with intellectual disabilities, the 'yellow book' (Stenfert Kroese et al. 1997), major steps have been taken to ensure that CBT is accessible to people with learning disabilities, offering them the same opportunities afforded to others who are suffering from emotional difficulties. Unfortunately, this simply isn't true. In this chapter we make a number of suggestions about what can be done to improve this situation.

One of the challenges of adapting interventions for different client groups is that therapies like CBT aren't static but are constantly evolving. This begs the question as to whether there is a risk that CBT for people with intellectual disabilities will always be one step behind mainstream work. Or is there a need to avoid making constant attempts to catch up with mainstream work before ensuring proper adaptations of existing approaches to CBT have been embedded in practice? That is not to say that innovations should be ignored. We have included a chapter in this book on mindfulness-based approaches and would not want people with intellectual disabilities to miss out on new developments in the field. Moreover, keeping abreast of developments is what helps to keep therapists engaged and enthusiastic in their work, a key ingredient of successful therapy. However, in our minds, there is no doubt that there is still a lot of fundamental work to be done to embed CBT in everyday practice with people who have intellectual disabilities.

The main aim of this chapter is to consider the systems and processes required to promote and sustain the use of CBT. Clearly, we are building on the training and supervisory frameworks used in general adult mental health, but we would like to make a case that what is required for people with intellectual disabilities isn't just a straightforward simplification. By using CBT with people who have intellectual disabilities, we have been forced to innovate and think critically about the underpinning theory and assumptions. By doing so, we believe that much has been added to the knowledge base of this field (even though that knowledge hasn't necessarily been communicated well to our colleagues in general adult mental health or always been taken seriously by them). For example, some of the key developments in anger management approaches were developed with people who have intellectual disabilities (Taylor et al. 2002), yet most people working in mental health would be unaware of this.

As therapists we have learned a great deal from the clients with intellectual disabilities we have worked with. While we recognise there is a major job to be done to develop processes and structures to support the delivery of CBT to people with intellectual disabilities, this should start with a conviction that the emotional lives of people with intellectual disabilities matter as much as anyone else's. Moreover, there should be a commitment to people with intellectual disabilities having access to the therapies that might help them.

General mental health professionals are often sceptical about the use of CBT with people who have intellectual disabilities, but arguments against using psychological therapies also come from those who support a social model of disability or who believe there needs to be more emphasis on a public health or health promotion model (Emerson and Hatton 2014). People with intellectual disabilities remain a marginalised and disenfranchised group and there is little sense that this is changing. One of the criticisms of psychological approaches like CBT is that they fail to address the underlying injustices faced by people with learning disabilities. Our view is that what we offer is not an 'either or' choice. We believe that therapists who are committed to people with intellectual disabilities need to be aware of the wider context of their lives. This might mean playing a proactive role in countering injustice and helping to foster opportunities for people to lead fulfilling lives. Equally, people with intellectual disabilities who experience emotional distress should have access to psychological therapies like CBT that have a strong evidence base supporting their use in the wider population. This means having therapists who are trained and have expertise in intellectual disabilities as well as in delivering therapies like CBT.

We would argue that limited access to psychological therapies is one example of the health inequalities faced by our clients (Emerson and Hatton 2014). Health inequalities are not a trivial matter and can be a matter of life or death. In a recent study in England examining the deaths of 244 people with intellectual disabilities, it was found that 28% of these deaths could have been prevented if good health care had been provided (Heslop et al. 2013). When it comes to mental health problems it would be unfair to suggest that therapists set out to be discriminatory. A more straightforward reason is that they often lack the know-how to provide sensitive support that meets the needs of clients with intellectual disabilities.

Why Train Therapists

At present there is no formal training available on delivering CBT to people with intellectual disabilities, beyond brief input to clinical psychology trainees in the UK. Therapists cannot be expected to develop the confidence and skills to use CBT on a routine basis with people who have intellectual disabilities, without training and supervision. Being left to adapt therapy as best they can leaves therapists wondering if they really are up to the mark or if what they are doing can really be called CBT. This need for specialised training has been recognised internationally (Man et al. 2016).

Dagnan et al. (2014) produced interesting findings from a survey of therapists about delivering psychological therapies to people with intellectual disabilities. Perhaps unsurprisingly, they found that prior training about people with intellectual disabilities and experience of delivering therapy to these clients were associated with greater confidence. A telling conclusion Dagnan et al. came to was that therapists who are well-equipped to work with people who have intellectual disabilities will also be better prepared to work with a much larger group of potential clients, who fall outside the category of intellectual disability but still have relatively low cognitive abilities. As shown below, whilst only 2% of the general population have an intellectual disability, 14% of the population have a borderline intellectual disability.

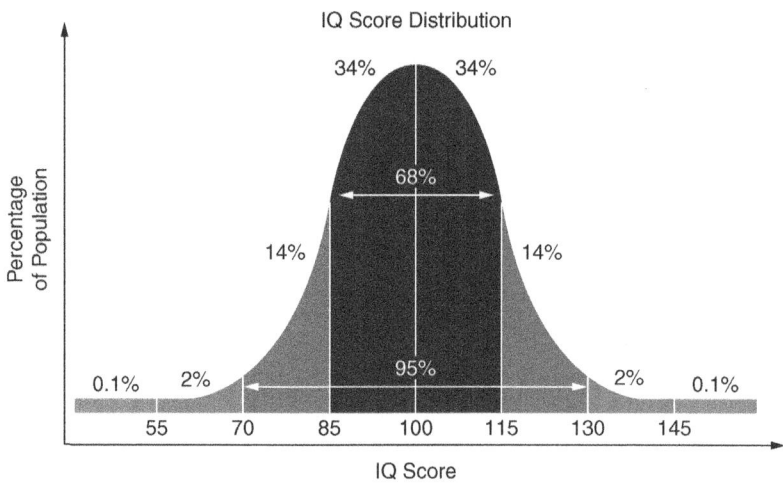

Thus, there is a large group of people with borderline difficulties who may also require adaptations to be able to benefit from CBT interventions.

Despite a lack of confidence, there is evidence to suggest that some therapists in specialist services might be doing a better job than they imagine with clients who have an intellectual disability. When we carried out research to examine key therapy process issues relating to the delivery of CBT to clients with an intellectual disability, one of the goals was to establish if we were actually delivering what might be considered to be CBT (Jahoda et al. 2009). As part of this study, 14 clients' sessions were rated using the cognitive therapy scale for psychosis (CTS-Psy; Haddock et al. 2001). It might seem strange to have selected a psychosis scale but we chose it because it comprehensively covers the content and processes that would be expected to be observed in a typical CBT session.

This includes looking at whether an agenda is completed and the therapist addresses key cognitions. From a process perspective, issues such as the use of a collaborative approach are part of the scale. Interestingly, the CTS also codes whether items are appropriately included, appropriately excluded or inappropriately excluded.

An overall score from 1 to 6 is given where the bottom of the scale is rated as 'a barely acceptable level of skill' and the top of the scale is 'an excellent level of skill' in terms of the therapist's CBT practice. Haddock et al. found that CBT therapists who were trained to a diploma level, which consists of a nine-month-long weekly training course, achieved a mean overall score of 2.2 out of a possible score of 6. Even though we regarded ourselves as CBT therapists, we were all rather anxious that we would be 'found out' when fidelity checks were completed by an experienced CBT trainer who was independent of those delivering the therapy. To our relief, all therapists showed fidelity to the model and of the overall ratings for the 14 sessions where CBT was carried out, one was rated at level 3 (satisfactory), eight were rated at level 4 (good) and five were rated as 5 (very good).

The detailed ratings carried out by the independent reviewer offered considerable food for thought, showing that therapists communicated well with clients and were largely successful in achieving collaborative relationships. There was also evidence that therapists worked on relevant cognitions and used 'guided discovery'. Perhaps unsurprisingly, some of the more complex questioning was less evident, like asking clients about the inconsistent conclusions they reach when talking about emotive events. Some typical elements of a CBT session were also often absent. For example, homework was only reviewed in half of the sessions that were rated. One straightforward interpretation of these findings is that it is more difficult to adapt more complicated aspects of therapy. Alternatively, perhaps some of the more complex elements of CBT were just too difficult for the clients involved in this study to grasp or use. These were all individuals with mild to moderate intellectual disabilities referred to specialist community mental health teams. So it may have been appropriate to modify these tasks or leave them out. Support available to clients beyond the therapy room also appeared key, as clients often needed help to complete homework tasks between sessions, which fits with our discussion of this issue (see Chaps. 4, 5 and 6).

The therapists' ratings in our study highlighted their core therapeutic skills and their ability to communicate well with the clients and develop a rapport. However, they appeared to struggle more with complex aspects of therapy, when it came to communicating about thoughts and feelings. Perhaps these are the key areas that specialist training for working with people who have intellectual disabilities should focus on.

A Framework for Specialist Training

The current vogue when talking about training for psychological therapies is to talk about 'competencies frameworks'. Essentially this means that therapists are trained to have the 'knowledge and skills' to deliver therapy to an expected standard for all client groups (Keen and Freeston 2008). The strength of using a competencies framework is that it helps to break down the particular knowledge and skills that therapists might need, including that gleamed from generic CBT training. For example, we know that the ability to generate a collaborative, non-judgemental approach and to take seriously people's perceptions of their world are greatly valued by clients with intellectual disabilities and are the foundations of CBT interventions (Pert et al. 2013). Generic training also teaches a range of specific skills including: (i) agenda setting, (ii) recording thoughts, feelings and behaviour, (iii) ways of questioning people about their perceptions of events and self, (iv) producing formulations, (v) ways of promoting more adaptive/compassionate ways of thinking, (vi) setting and completing homework tasks, (vii) behavioural techniques such as relaxation training. Higher level skills tend to concern what works for whom, linked to the formulation. Moreover, there are specific approaches which are linked to theories about particular presenting difficulties.

Throughout this book we have tried to consider (i) how people with intellectual disabilities' cognitive difficulties might have an impact on how they engage with CBT—as a talking therapy communication remains key, (ii) the person's phenomenology, or how their self and interpersonal perceptions might be shaped by their particular experience, and (iii) the importance of taking account of the broader context of the person's life if change is to be achieved and maintained. Consequently, perhaps the best place to start when training CBT therapists who are going to work with clients who have an intellectual disability is with the person. Therapists need to know who people with intellectual disabilities are and the sense CBT is likely to make, when considered in the broader context of their lives. Moreover, the therapists need to grasp the challenges to engagement in therapy that difficulties with expressive and receptive communication, memory, planning and other cognitive problems might pose. This leads into a consideration of key adaptations concerning (i) process, (ii) the use of materials, (iii) key techniques and (iv) adopting a collaborative approach with significant others and fellow professionals. Of course, these elements are not mutually exclusive but overlap. For example, overcoming communication barriers might have implications for choosing which materials are used and the need to involve others to support the client.

There are clearly core skills and techniques that remain the same, whoever the therapist is working with, but additional training with regard to communication skills is an important area. As stated in Chaps. 4, 5 and 6, this goes beyond the therapist's facility to simplify language. It is also about being comfortable with idiosyncratic styles of communication and helping clients to remain engaged, whilst at the same time ensuring clients feel like they are being listened to and have an active role to play in sessions. Therapists also need to know how to adapt existing materials and find more accessible materials. Other more specific skills might include teaching and supporting clients to complete self-report forms or how to master therapeutic exercises like relaxation training. Being prepared for the possible involvement of significant others in the client's life yet respecting confidentiality and knowing how to work collaboratively on aspects of therapy are also important skills. Tackling stigma and disadvantage can be key aspects of a therapeutic intervention and may require the therapist to play a more active role in supporting change outside a therapeutic setting than would ordinarily be the case.

There needs to be some caution when advocating a competence-based approach. Whilst the aim is to ensure that therapists reach an acceptable level, being competent does not necessarily mean that you are a good therapist (Fairburn and Cooper 2011). In some ways, competency frameworks for therapy remind us of past research one of us was involved in concerning the quality of care for people with intellectual disabilities. Introducing inspections or ways of monitoring care are effective in reducing bad or substandard practice and ensuring reasonable standards are maintained. The risk is that they demand conformity to a reasonable standard and can have the unintended effect of stifling innovative and excellent practice. When working with clients who might need a creative approach to engage with them and overcome communicative and other barriers, care has to be taken to ensure that therapists' creative spark isn't extinguished. It would be wrong to think that creativity is the antithesis of a scientist-practitioner model, as described in the section on metacompetence at the end of Chap. 3.

If it proves impossible to keep a client on track in sessions, when using guided discovery to elicit and discuss their cognitions, then the therapist may decide to try a different approach. For example, to avoid the client becoming preoccupied with particular tangential events, the therapist might try using stories about another person, to help the client consider different ways of thinking about and responding to the situation. For example, a client with significant anger problems may have a tendency to go off on tangents in therapy sessions when talking about situations of conflict. Consequently, the therapist might take an alternative tack of talking about another person who has similar anger problems, to help the client consider different ways of thinking about and responding to conflict. We have a series of films about situations of conflict that clients enjoy working with. Whether such an approach is successful or not can be determined by observing if the client does indeed remain on task and if it allows him or her to consider different perspectives. Creative approaches can be both rigorous and person centred.

Materials and Supervision

Of course, just because people have been trained doesn't mean that they actually use their training. An important question to ask is whether therapists who have been trained to deliver CBT to people who have intellectual disabilities actually go on to use this approach in their day-to-day work? One group of professionals who commonly receive some limited training about how to adapt CBT for people with intellectual disabilities are clinical psychologists. Although we don't have data about the number of clinical psychologists working in specialist health services for people with intellectual disabilities in the UK who use CBT on a regular basis, anecdotally the number appears to be surprisingly small. A researcher, who was recently looking for clinicians delivering CBT to people with intellectual disabilities in a large service with more than 15 full-time psychologists, could only find two who said they were using CBT with clients. Similarly, when we carried out our research examining process issues in delivering CBT to clients with intellectual disabilities it proved a major challenge to find sufficient numbers of therapists who were using CBT with clients on a regular basis (Jahoda et al. 2009).

One reason that clinical psychologists may not be using CBT with clients who have an intellectual disability is because their training has been inadequate. However, we strongly suspect that this is not the only reason. Learning how to deliver CBT means being supervised to deliver therapy to a range of people with intellectual disabilities and gaining direct experience of overcoming communicative and other barriers. Having a limited number of people delivering CBT to people with intellectual disabilities means there will be little peer support available for therapists and little opportunity for more formal supervision of practice. So there may be a vicious circle, whereby the lack of support available for CBT therapists (whether clinical psychologists or not) means that few of them maintain or capitalise on the training they have, resulting in a failure to build a critical mass of competent and confident therapists who can train others.

Increasing Access and the Mainstreaming Debate

One way forward might be to equip CBT therapists working in mainstream services with the skills to provide appropriate and sensitive input for people with intellectual disabilities. Internationally, there are many countries that lack specialist services for people with intellectual disabilities, so this is the only route open to them. There are also calls for people with intellectual disabilities to have access to mainstream services for more positive reasons such as gaining access to therapists who have real expertise in CBT and having the opportunity to use the same services as everyone else. However, the willingness and ability of mainstream therapists to address the needs of people with intellectual disabilities remains a matter of contention.

As described in Chap. 2, this shift to mainstream services is meant to be happening in an English initiative called 'Increasing Access for Psychological Therapies' (IAPT). This service is meant to be open to all, offering equal access to different client groups experiencing mental health problems. IAPT leans heavily on the use of CBT approaches. However, as is often the case, there appears to be a gap between the rhetoric and the reality. For one thing accessing the service can be difficult, in part because it is based on a system of self-referral, which, as we have already mentioned, rarely happens with people who have intellectual disabilities (Chinn and Abraham 2016). Moreover, the manualised materials have been developed for people using general adult mental health services and require literacy skills. The service effectiveness is also closely monitored and that involves clients having to complete a large number of self-report questionnaires on a regular basis. Once again, these questionnaires rely on clients having literacy skills and being able to make sense of complex items. IAPT services thus face a significant challenge in terms of adapting materials for people with intellectual disabilities. Not only that, they are also penalised if the self-report questionnaires are not completed. Beyond these bureaucratic barriers, using strictly manualised and time-limited interventions makes it difficult to slow down the pace of sessions and adapt the approach for particular clients' needs. Thus, there would seem to be few incentives for therapists and their managers to make their service flexible enough to meet the psychological needs of people with intellectual disabilities (Chinn and Abraham 2016).

The news from IAPT isn't all negative. There are examples of exciting local initiatives to train therapists to adapt CBT therapy materials, loosen up the rigid manuals and time frames, with training for staff to deliver interventions to people with intellectual disabilities (Dagnan et al. 2015).

These initiatives rely on supervision and support from local specialist intellectual disability services. Consequently, there is an opportunity to build bridges with mainstream services for people with intellectual disabilities. As stated previously, developing more accessible, engaging and flexible CBT therapeutic approaches would also be to the advantage of less able clients more generally, who also often suffer from health inequalities (Dagnan et al. 2014).

Manuals: Mapping a Way Ahead

The more positive experience of the IAPT well-being therapists suggests that a possible way forward in delivering CBT to people with intellectual disabilities would be the development of more straightforward CBT manuals, offering a clear framework for dealing with particular emotional difficulties clients might have. Therapists have a real thirst for relevant materials they can use and guidance about what to do. We have spoken in previous chapters, particularly with regard to group work, about the use of existing manuals. Having a structured approach offers a solid framework for the training and supervision of therapists. You can keep track of whether someone has followed an approach properly or not and delivering a set of sessions on a regular basis means that the therapist can become practised at delivering the intervention. Familiarity might also make it easier to bring the materials to life for individual clients. Manuals could contain hints and tips about overcoming common barriers.

For most therapists it's a great comfort to know what they need to do in sessions and to be provided with tried and tested ideas that actually seem to work. For example, Paul Willner's (Willner et al. 2013) anger management manual includes a number of engaging exercises, like shaking up a bottle of fizzy water, to illustrate what happens when people's arousal builds and they lose their temper. Although most existing manuals have been developed for group work there are also a number of manuals developed for individual CBT that we have mentioned in the course of the book (Taylor and Novaco 2005; Hassiotis et al. 2013; Lindsay et al. 2015). A final advantage of manualised approaches is that they are more straightforward to evaluate, helping to build an evidence base about the effectiveness of CBT approaches with people who have intellectual disabilities.

Manuals may not always prove successful. A trans-diagnostic CBT manual was developed by Hassiotis et al. (2013), to address problems of anxiety, depression and anger. The manual is described as being suitable for therapists with little or no previous experience of delivering therapy to people with intellectual disabilities. However, the pilot randomised controlled trial of the manual showed little evidence of effectiveness, in terms of reducing self-reported symptoms of distress. While this was a pilot study and a host of factors might explain the findings, it still raises the question about the training and supervision that therapists require to operationalise a manual of this nature. A transdiagnostic manual evaluated by Lindsay et al. (2015), in a specialist service, fared better.

Of course, manuals have their critics and are often considered too restrictive. Unless clients find the intervention engaging and relevant, the therapy is unlikely to be helpful. Moreover, not all clients' problems can be neatly diagnosed to fit with manuals for particular emotional difficulties like anxiety, depression or anger, with the risk that a client feels misunderstood rather than helped. However, manuals don't have to be restrictive and can have the scope to be more or less flexible and sensitive, in terms of content, length and the potential to address individual needs. Whatever the drawbacks, developing a broader range of suitable CBT materials, manuals and guidance for working with people who have intellectual disabilities is a vital step towards instilling greater confidence and purpose amongst therapists. To find out the best way of using these materials, there should also be research concerning the relative effectiveness of supervised delivery of CBT manuals compared with unsupervised therapists who take them off the shelf and give them a go.

Broadening Access to CBT

Another approach to increasing access to CBT for people with intellectual disabilities is to train a broader range of therapists, including lay therapists, to deliver interventions to people with intellectual disabilities. As Chap. 6 shows, there are already a number of group-based interventions designed to be delivered to people with an intellectual disability by health or social care professionals trained to act as therapists. In fact, it may already be the case in the UK that people with an intellectual disability are most likely to encounter CBT in the form of an anger management or anxiety management group run by health or social care professionals.

We were recently involved in a randomised control trial of an anger management intervention delivered by lay therapists who were social care staff working in day services (Willner et al. 2013; see Chap. 6 for more details). The sessions run by the therapists were coded for fidelity, to find out how well the lay therapists followed and delivered the manualised intervention. The rating scale developed for this purpose was called the Manualised Group Intervention Checklist, and given the unassuming acronym of MAGIC (Jahoda et al. 2013; see www.toolsfortalking.wordpress.com). The checklist included items about how well the therapists managed the group and engaged the clients in the therapeutic process. A particular strength of the lay therapists proved to be their communication skills. Generally, they were also conscientious about delivering the manual, carrying out the set activities and making appropriate use of the materials. Where they were weakest was in covering the more complex CBT elements and talking with the clients who took part about their thoughts and feelings. Unfortunately, the training and manual did not appear to give the lay therapists a sufficient grasp of the relevant theory or the necessary therapeutic skills to cover these key CBT components.

Of course, like all large-scale studies, the descriptive data provide an overview of what happened. Direct observation of sessions revealed stark differences in the abilities of the lay therapists. Some did a remarkable job of delivering the sessions, running the group with panache whilst remaining sensitive to particular needs of different group members. Other lay therapists were remote and unimaginative or failed to grasp the purpose of the sessions. So it would be wrong to dismiss the use of lay therapists altogether but care needs to be taken when selecting therapists and perhaps an instrument like MAGIC could be used to help identify those more suited to this role.

A metacompetency-based strategy for delivering CBT tends to follow the logic that the more skilled a therapist you are, the more complex cases you are able to deal with. And to a large extent that is what we are suggesting here, the use of social and health care professionals with experience of working with people who have intellectual disabilities, who are given a short training to deliver a specific manualised intervention, supervised by more experienced and better trained CBT therapists. However, we need to exercise a little care over this kind of approach for several reasons. Firstly, simplistic ideas about the assessed complexity of individual difficulties fail to take account of the dynamic nature of people's lives. While some individuals thankfully overcome serious emotional problems without significant input, other people's difficulties stubbornly fail to improve or deteriorate unexpectedly. The risk is that clients will be expected to fit into the structure of specific CBT interventions, rather than the service being flexible enough to meet the changing needs of clients.

Another potential flaw of a stepped care model is the assumption that the most highly trained CBT therapists should only work with those who present with the most significant problems. Yet if these highly trained therapists are to have credibility when they're supervising less well-trained therapists, then they need to be familiar with interventions their supervisees are delivering. Moreover, it could also be argued that sometimes clients with complex difficulties are not going to be in a state of mind to respond to the most complex type of CBT interventions and may benefit more from more contained and straightforward approaches. The therapist's skill might not relate to the level of complex intervention they can deliver but more to knowing about what kind of intervention might be best suited to the client's needs.

We would advocate a model where the more highly trained CBT therapists provide supervision for therapists delivering lower level manualised approaches. However, throughout this book we have argued for the need for a creative approach and for therapy to be meaningful for clients; hence the supervisors need to have a continuing grasp of how to deliver the materials in practice and how they can be tailored to individual needs. Even the most experienced clinician requires ongoing supervision to ensure good practice and those working with clients who have intellectual disabilities are no exception.

Conclusion

Most of this book has concerned ways of adapting and making CBT relevant for people with intellectual disabilities and how it can be best delivered to individuals and groups. However, a major issue for people with intellectual disabilities is getting access to psychological therapies like CBT in the first place. In services there's a lot of talk about implementation science and, whether we use this jargon or not, there does seem to be a need for research on how best to build an infrastructure that delivers CBT to people with intellectual disabilities most effectively. Another potential arena to explore is the online community. Electronic media makes it far easier for a dispersed group of therapists to share ideas and to seek advice than was previously the case. It is with this in mind that we have created a website for some of our 'home-made' materials (www.toolsfortalking.wordpress.com). There might be value in developing a virtual community to bring together therapists, share materials and ideas and even link up new CBT therapists with experienced practitioners. In turn, this could be linked to the possibilities of harnessing technological developments to assist with the delivery of CBT for people with intellectual disabilities. We need to ensure that people with intellectual disabilities benefit from these developments.

> **Key Points**
> - There is a need to broaden people with intellectual disabilities' access to psychological services for people with intellectual disabilities.
> - Whilst there may be a shift to the delivery of CBT to people with intellectual disabilities by mainstream services, there remains a need for some specialist support and training.
> - Thought needs to be given to a more systematic approach to the training and supervision of therapists delivering CBT.
> - Where therapy is delivered by lay therapists then supervision is essential.
> - Adapted manuals and materials should be made more freely available.
> - Electronic media provide an opportunity to build on online community of more dispersed CBT therapists and a means of offering peer support both nationally and internationally.

References

Chinn, D., & Abraham, E. (2016). Using 'candidacy' as a framework for understanding access to mainstream psychological treatment for people with intellectual disabilities and common mental health problems within the English improving access to psychological therapies service. *Journal of Intellectual Disabilities Research, 60,* 571–582.

Dagnan, D., Masson, J., Cavagin, A., Thwaites, R., & Hatton, C. (2014). The development of a measure of confidence in delivering therapy to people with intellectual disabilities. *Clinical Psychology & Psychotherapy, 22,* 392–398.

Dagnan, D., Burke, C.-K., Davies, J., & Chinn, D. (2015). *Improving access to psychological therapies: Learning disabilities positive practice guide.* London: Foundation for People with Learning Disabilities.

Emerson, E., & Hatton, C. (2014). *Health inequalities and people with intellectual disabilities.* Cambridge: Cambridge University Press.

Fairburn, C. G., & Cooper, Z. (2011). Therapist competence, therapy quality, and therapist training. *Behaviour Research and Therapy, 49,* 373–378.

Haddock, G., Devane, S., Bradshaw, T., McGovern, J., Tarrier, N., Kinderman, P., Baguley, I., Lancashire, S., & Harris, N. (2001). An investigation into the psychometric properties of the cognitive therapy scale for psychosis (CTS-Psy). *Behavioural and Cognitive Psychotherapy, 29,* 221–233.

Hassiotis, A., Serfaty, M., Azam, K., Strydom, A., Martin, S., Parkes, C., Blizard, R., et al. (2013). Manualised Individual Cognitive Behavioural Therapy for mood disorders in people with mild to moderate intellectual disability: A feasibility randomised controlled trial. *Journal of Affective Disorders, 151*(1), 186–195.

Heslop, P., Blair, P., Fleming, P., Hoghton, M., Marriott, A., & Russ, L. (2013). The confidential inquiry into premature deaths of people with intellectual disabilities in the UK: A population-based study. *The Lancet,* 62026–62027. doi:10.1016/S0140-6736. (published online).

Jahoda, A., Selkirk, M., Trower, P., Pert, C., Stenfert Kroese, B., Dagnan, D., & Burford, B. (2009). The balance of power in therapeutic interactions with individuals who have intellectual disabilities. *British Journal of Clinical Psychology, 48*(1), 63–77. ISSN 0144-6657.

Jahoda, A., Willner, P., Rose, J., Stenfert Kroese, B., Felce, D., Cohen, D., MacMahon, P., Stimpson, A., Rose, N., Gillespie, D., Shead, J., Lammie, C., Woodgate, C., Townson, J., Nuttall, J., & Hood, K. (2013). Development of a scale to measure fidelity to manualized group-based cognitive behavioural interventions for people with intellectual disabilities. *Research in Developmental Disabilities, 34*, 4210–42221.

Keen, A. J., & Freeston, M. H. (2008). Assessing competence in cognitive-behavioural therapy. *British Journal of Psychiatry, 193*, 60–64.

Lindsay, W. R., Tinsley, S., Beail, N., Hastings, R. P., Jahoda, A., Taylor, J. L., & Hatton, C. (2015). A preliminary controlled trial of a trans-diagnostic programme for cognitive behaviour therapy with adults with intellectual disability. *Journal of Intellectual Disability Research, 59*(4), 360–369. doi:10.1111/jir.12145.

Man, J., Kangas, M., Trollor, J., & Sweller, N. (2016). Clinical competencies and training needs of psychologists working with adults with intellectual disability and co-morbid mental ill health. *Clinical Psychologist.* doi:10.1111/cp.12092 _ USE THIS. Advance online publication.

Pert, C., Jahoda, A., Stenfert Kroese, B., Trower, P., Dagnan, D., & Selkirk, M. (2013). Cognitive behavioural therapy from the perspective of clients with mild intellectual disabilities: A qualitative investigation of process issues. *Journal of Intellectual Disability Research, 57*, 359–369. doi:10.1111/j.1365-2788.2012.01546.x.

Stenfert Kroese, B., Dagnan, D., & Loumidis, K. (Eds.). (1997). *Cognitive-behaviour therapy for people with learning disabilities* (pp. 110–123). London: Routledge.

Taylor, J. L., & Novaco, R. W. (2005). *Anger treatment for people with developmental disabilities: A theory, evidence and manual based approach*. Chichester: Wiley.

Taylor, J. L., Novaco, R. W., Gillmer, B., & Thorne, I. (2002). Cognitive-behavioural treatment of anger intensity among offenders with intellectual disabilities. *Journal of Applied Research in Intellectual Disabilities, 15*, 151–165.

Willner, P., Rose, J., Jahoda, A., Stenfert Kroese, B., Felce, D., Cohen, D., MacMahon, P., Stimpson, A., Rose, N., Gillespie, D., Shead, J., Lammie, C., Woodgate, C., Townson, J., Nuttall, J., & Hood, K. (2013). Outcomes of a cluster-randomized controlled trial of a group-based cognitive behavioural anger management intervention for people with mild to moderate intellectual disabilities. *British Journal of Psychiatry., 203*, 288–296.

12

Final Thoughts

Looking back over the process of writing this book together, we are aware that despite our efforts to collect, comprehend and disseminate a large amount of clinical and academic knowledge and experience in CBT for people with intellectual disabilities, we remain in a position of 'informed ignorance' and still have a lot to learn. We would have liked to cover more topics such as transition to adulthood and being a parent with an intellectual disability, and some topics that have been mentioned (such as sexuality, autism and bereavement) in much more detail. However, we hope that by putting together our efforts so far, the reader is able to gain something from our limited knowledge and experience or at least is inspired to begin or continue their own journey of discovery. To end this book, we present a few final thoughts.

There has been an explosion of interest in the biological basis of behaviour. In his last term in office, President Obama announced his Brain Initiative, with a huge investment into neuropsychology, including an explicit attempt to obtain greater understanding of developmental difficulties like autism. In the field of intellectual disability there has also been an increasing focus on understanding the behavioural phenotypes of different genetic syndromes and developmental difficulties, a welcome acknowledgement that people with intellectual disabilities are not a homogeneous group (Waite et al. 2014). CBT therapists will find it helpful to have new insights into the effects of particular cognitive impairments on how people interpret events and act. For example, there has been important progress in tailoring CBT interventions for people with autism (Lang et al. 2010). However, if there are too many different adaptations of CBT for different developmental disabilities, then there is a risk that the approach will become fragmented. In turn, it could become difficult to train and support therapists to deliver CBT to people with intellectual disabilities.

A concern with the brain needs to be matched by an abiding concern with the common humanity of people with intellectual disabilities. Of course, the strength of a CBT approach is that it involves developing a formulation for each client that is based on their individual history, characteristics including their strengths and their presenting problems. This is in contrast to a pathological diagnostic approach which attempts to fit the client in a specific category. CBT allows us to consider the uniqueness of our clients and makes us more likely to consider them as people rather than as mere problems. For example, a CBT formulation will focus on *what* a person with autistic features is thinking over and above *how* they think.

An emerging view about people who have autism is that different developmental trajectories should not always be thought of as disability but as a different way of relating to the world that should be celebrated rather than 'fixed' (Silberman 2015). While this view does not tend to be applied to people with an intellectual disability because they are thought to lack the very particular strengths of people with autism (e.g. above-average memory function and non-verbal intelligence), we would argue that embracing and respecting difference has to be the cornerstone of working as a CBT therapist with people who have intellectual disabilities. If a therapist fails to accept people for who they are, then how is that therapist going to help them to feel good about themselves? This is why we have stressed throughout this book the importance of a strong therapeutic relationship and paid particular attention to process issues in therapy. For example, in Chap. 5 we refer to the Westbrook et al. (2010) model that focuses on the interface between client characteristics and therapist characteristics, including their values and attitudes. Such an approach helps us to look beyond our concerns with client 'deficits' and focus on the interpersonal aspects of the therapeutic encounter.

Of course, developmental difficulties can have subtle effects on how people interact with the world. For example, if someone struggles to adjust to change then those offering support might quite understandably make efforts to protect the person from disruption by, for example, adhering to rigid household routines and shielding them from disturbing or unexpected news. While this might be a successful way of accommodating the person's particular difficulties, in the long term this might make change even more anxiety provoking and distressing because the person has failed to develop strategies for coping with change.

People's lives are complicated and having an intellectual disability does not make a person's life less complicated. We have tried to get the point across in this book that there may not always be a simple or right answer when it comes to helping someone to use a therapeutic approach like CBT. One of the first ideas that we talked about was the influence of George Kelly on the development of CBT (1977). He argued that in clinical work it is important to start with an understanding of the person, rather than trying to fit the person to the theory. In this book we have tried to start with the person with an intellectual disability and think about how CBT can be applied to his or her particular circumstances.

What often emerges when we teach mental health professionals about the challenges of adapting CBT for people with intellectual disabilities are concerns and questions about the core ideas underlying the approach. For example, how do you work to achieve change with people who have limited control over their lives or how do you build a collaborative relationship with people whose usual relationships with professionals are subordinate ones? A common response from students and staff is to say that these issues are not unique to people with intellectual disabilities. They go on to talk about sometimes facing similar difficulties in general adult mental health settings, when working with people who are poor, socially marginalised or who are disempowered for other reasons. We hope that many of the ideas discussed in this book may also be helpful when delivering CBT to other populations.

As therapists, we have brought different perspectives and interests to this book. I would like to say that we had fierce discussions when we met in the

Bashful Alley café in Lancaster for our book meetings, but we were too preoccupied with the tea and cake for that. Nevertheless, we have negotiated areas of difference, including the use of terms like 'metacompetence'. Whatever language was used in the different chapters, our common goal has been to highlight the need for therapists to have the ability to creatively adapt CBT for people with intellectual disabilities. Another core idea in this book is the need for therapists to take account of the broader context of the person's life seriously when formulating and working with their emotional difficulties. We recognise that involving other people to the extent that we have suggested in previous chapters might stretch the traditional understanding of the CBT model. Consequently, it might be fair to say that we have proposed an enhanced or contextualised type of CBT.

Taking account of clients' lives and broader circumstances is not just for pragmatic reasons, nor does it mean abandoning theory for a 'feel good' approach. On the contrary, we have tried to emphasise the need for theory to underpin the suggested adaptations. In particular, we have pointed to the work of Vygotsky and the zone of proximal development to help promote an understanding of how working in partnership with others and 'scaffolding' can help clients achieve more than if they were working on their own (Reiber and Robinson 2004). This is a particularly important idea when individual cognitive impairments might limit what clients can achieve alone. Moreover, symbolic interactionism provides a rationale for working alongside significant others in a client's life, in an effort to help shift clients' self and interpersonal perceptions (Jahoda et al. 2009). This is consistent with the notion that clients learn through their active engagement with the world, as well as through therapeutic dialogue and introspection.

In addition to being therapists, all of us are actively involved in research, and we would strongly advocate the need for further research to underpin the adaptations to CBT we have suggested. We are not just talking about carrying out major outcome trials, although that would be good. It would also be useful to explore key process issues, such as the most effective way of involving significant others in the therapeutic process with clients. Are shared formulations helpful and do role plays lead to the desired shift in clients' perspectives? Then there are the bigger questions. CBT is a multi-element approach and it would be immensely helpful to have a better idea about the active ingredients for people with intellectual disabilities. In other words, if the therapist knew what aspects of therapy are most accessible and useful to people with intellectual disabilities, then they would also have a better idea about where and how to focus their efforts. Not all of this needs to be high-level research; good case studies can make telling contribution to the literature. What we need is a commitment from researchers as well as from 'scientist-practitioners' to build an evidence base to support and improve the delivery of CBT to people with an intellectual disability. This means that as well as large-scale funded research studies conducted by university researchers, CBT practitioners share their experiences with others by publishing or presenting case studies whenever they consider their CBT techniques to be particularly successful (or not at all) and discuss and drill deeper to find out the reasons for this.

In order to retain a keen sense of discovery (not always easy in the day-to-day reality of working in isolation with little opportunity to share ideas, dealing with heavy caseloads and the pressure to deal with clients quickly and efficiently), we must pay attention to our own developmental and psychological needs. That is, we must allow ourselves time to think and to learn, not just as students and trainees, but throughout our careers. Post-qualification training and reading is essential to keep a fresh perspective, as is regular clinical supervision.

As therapists, we think that one of the most important attributes to have and to maintain is a sense of curiosity. Curiosity about people, how they function, their strengths and interests and why things do not always go well for them. We have found that when working with people with intellectual disabilities, this curiosity is easily preserved because our clients often have original and creative ways of dealing with their world. But trying to find out why someone hides food and small objects under their mattress or refuses to speak to anyone (or both!) can be a very complex task and we don't pretend that our methods can ever reveal a person's thinking and functioning in all its complexities.

When Hamlet realises he is being manipulated by family and friends, he asks one of the culprits, his supposed friend Guildenstern, to pick up a simple flute and play a melody. Guildenstern replies that he has never played a flute in his life and has no idea how to. Hamlet scorns him and points out that he has the arrogance to think that he can 'play' him

(Hamlet) yet is baffled by such a very simple flute: 'You would seem to know my stops. You would pluck out the heart of my mystery ... do you think I am easier to be played on than a pipe?' (Act 3, Scene 2).

Unlike Guildenstern, we are very aware that our CBT formulations are often no more than tentative hypotheses that may or may not reflect at least some of the ways in which our clients deal with their environments. We would never pretend to fully understand another person's psychological functioning. Yet attempting to gain some insight into our clients' ways of thinking, although challenging on many levels, we know, can be helpful and result in positive consequences. It requires empathy, creativity as well as curiosity on the part of the therapist. The late Herb Lovett (Lovett 2002) called his excellent book on working with people with difficult behaviour *Learning to Listen*, a phrase that resonates for us and reminds us that a skilled therapist first and foremost tunes into the messages sent by the client, be they verbal or not, and respectfully and carefully considers these messages before coming to any conclusions.

In the end, we come back to the importance of core values and the rights of people with intellectual disabilities. The notion of therapeutic disdain arose from the idea that therapists were not only sceptical about the ability of people with an intellectual disability to benefit from CBT but they also considered these individuals unworthy of their therapeutic skills (Bender 1993). In our view, we are perhaps at a different stage now, at least in the UK. Few CBT therapists are likely to show disdain for people with intellectual disabilities but they may lack the confidence and knowledge to work with people with an intellectual disability. The next step is to equip the therapists with the know-how they require.

References

Bender, M. (1993). The unoffered chair: The history of therapeutic disdain towards people with a learning difficulty. *Clinical Psychology Forum, 54*, 7–12.

Jahoda, A., Dagnan, D., Stenfert Kroese, B., Pert, C., & Trower, P. (2009). Cognitive behavioural therapy: From face to face interaction to a broader contextual understanding of change. *Journal of Intellectual Disability Research, 53*, 759–771.

Kelly, G. A. (1977). Personal construct theory and the psychotherapeutic interview. *Cognitive Therapy and Research, 1*(4), 355–362.

Lang, R., Regester, A., Lauderdale, S., Ashbaugh, K., & Haring, A. (2010). Treatment of anxiety in autism spectrum disorders using cognitive behaviour therapy: A systematic review. *Developmental Neurorehabilitation, 13*(1), 53–63.

Lovett, H. (2002). *Learning to listen – Positive approaches and people with difficult behavior* (4th ed.). Baltimore: Brookes.

Reiber, R. W., & Robinson, D. K. (Eds.). (2004). *The essential Vygotsky*. New York: Plenum.

Silberman, S. (2015). *Neurotribes: The legacy of autism and how to think smarter about people who think differently*. NSW: Allen and Unwin.

Waite, J., Heald, M., Wilde, L., Woodcock, K., Welham, A., Adams, D., et al. (2014). The importance of understanding the behavioural phenotypes of genetic syndromes associated with intellectual disability. *Paediatrics and Child Health, 24*, 468–472. doi:10.1016/j.paed.2014.05.002.

Westbrook, D., Mueller, M., Kennerley, H., & McManus, F. (2010). Common problems in therapy. In M. Mueller, H. Kennerley, F. McManus, & D. Westbrook (Eds.), *The Oxford guide to surviving as a CBT therapist*. Oxford: Oxford University Press.

Index

A

abstract concepts, 141, 196, 197
abuse, 20, 21, 33, 101, 171, 220
acceptance, 101, 128, 160, 161, 185–91, 193, 194, 200
Acceptance and Commitment Therapy, 10, 181, 183
accessible formulation, 103, 146–9
adaptive functioning, 216, 231
agency, 16, 22, 112, 113, 127, 133, 222
agenda, 32, 64, 111, 139, 140, 174, 175, 241, 242
aggression, 18, 33, 34, 68, 96, 102, 143, 144, 147, 148, 152, 183, 202, 219
agoraphobia, 61, 96
anger
 control, 159, 198
 management, 15, 23, 97, 102, 121, 134, 170, 172, 222, 238, 247, 249

Anger Inventory, 70
anxiety management, 249
Applied Behaviour Analysis, 3
appraisals, 17, 37, 95, 128, 142, 144–7, 150, 154
artful delivery, 47
assertiveness, 144
assessment, 5, 38, 44–6, 55–82, 89–91, 93, 124, 145, 153, 154, 217, 221, 224
attention, 5, 11, 16, 17, 24, 41, 45, 61, 66, 73, 87, 104, 112, 122, 137, 139, 154, 155, 159, 164, 168, 169, 177, 183–9, 195, 198–202, 256, 259
 control, 200
 span, 47, 173
attitudes
 cultural, 214
 negative, 214, 226
 social, 214

autistic spectrum disorder (ASD), 32
  Asperger's, 123
  autism, 120, 123, 255, 256
automatic pilot, 187, 188, 198, 199
automatic thoughts, 11, 18
avoidance, 189, 190
awareness, 5, 16, 21, 35, 58, 125, 168, 184–9, 191, 195, 197–201, 206, 215

B

bar charts, 77
behaviour
  adaptive, 12, 16, 160, 227, 242
  challenging, 32, 33, 72, 159, 227
behavioural experiments, 12, 38, 158
bereavement, 19, 97, 255
body awareness, 186, 187
body scan, 186, 187
Brief Symptom Inventory, 71
bullying, 21, 33, 124, 147, 148, 150, 215, 227
burn out, 226
Butler Self Image Profile, 79

C

case study, 5, 137, 142
catastrophising, 11, 122, 128
catchphrases, 189, 197
centred, 161
challenging behaviour, 33, 72, 159, 230
choice, 32, 35, 58, 78, 140, 141, 218, 220, 223, 229, 233, 238
client-centred, vi, 160, 161
clinical psychologists, 2, 60, 62, 159, 245

cognitions, 12, 34, 38, 44, 45, 68–70, 94, 96, 99, 102, 117, 190, 241, 244
cognitive, 44
  deficits, 15, 16, 26, 46, 68, 154
  distortions, 15–17, 26
  mediating events, 218
  mediation, 43–5, 66
  restructuring techniques, 192
  rigidity, 142, 146, 153, 154
  therapeutic strategies, 13
  Therapy Scale for Psychosis (CTS-psy), 240
collaborative empiricism, 37
collaborative relationship, 42, 116, 227, 257
comfort, 171, 194, 196, 203, 205, 247
commitment therapy, 183
communication
  poor, 229
  skills, 41, 173, 243, 249
communities, 14, 21, 37, 153, 215, 216, 222, 228, 231, 232, 241, 251
community nurses, 113, 231
community psychology, 214, 215
compassion, 184, 185, 188, 193–5, 202–5
Compassion Focussed Therapy (CFT), 10, 181, 184, 193, 195, 207
compassionate image, 194, 202–4
compensation, 46, 49
competence inhibiting support, 48, 61
competence promoting support, 48, 61
comprehension, 38, 39, 47, 140, 231

computerised training, 45
confidentiality, 58, 61, 217, 218, 220, 224, 226, 233, 243
consent, 153, 169, 221
context, 1, 5, 18, 20–2, 25, 31–49, 58, 62, 70, 87–9, 99, 100, 105, 127, 153, 158, 166, 167, 172, 182, 184, 193, 196, 226, 239, 243, 258
coping, 162
coping skills/strategies, 33, 43, 123, 152, 159, 162, 167, 168, 174, 176, 214, 215, 217, 221, 222, 226
core beliefs, 11, 145, 147
CORE-LD, 71
co-therapist, 158, 217
creative, vi, vii, 1, 82, 109–11, 118, 134, 137, 207, 244, 250, 259
cue cards, 138, 140, 141, 151, 192, 196
culture, 21, 218, 227

D

decentering, 191, 192, 199
dependency, 33, 40, 41, 65
depression, 10, 11, 13–15, 33, 34, 40, 73, 95, 96, 100, 101, 134, 158, 162, 163, 182–4, 219, 248
diagnostic
  classifications, 21, 232
  model, 232
  overshadowing, 36
  reliability and validity, 232
Dialectical Behaviour Therapy, 181, 183, 196
diaries, 4, 60, 71–5, 82, 138, 143, 153, 172, 173, 226

dichotomous thinking, 144
disabilities
  physical, 33, 205, 214
  sensory, 214
distractibility, 137, 139, 140
distributed competence, 48
DSM-V, 21

E

emotion recognition, 41
emotional
  exhaustion, 226
  intelligence, 35
  problems, 20, 21, 61, 67, 96, 117, 133, 250
  support, 100, 143, 222
  well-being, 99, 117
empathy, 42, 68, 99, 153, 155, 161, 260
engagement, 15, 45, 58, 67, 79, 89, 116, 119, 123, 138, 140, 148, 154, 160, 243, 258
environment(s)
  community, 231
  home, 171
  work, 48, 231
Equality Act, 31
evaluative beliefs, 91, 145
executive functioning, 41, 72, 230
expectations, 15, 56, 58, 82, 88, 126, 189, 190, 217, 218
externalising, 149, 219, 220

F

family
  care, 215, 216
  centred, 216

family (cont.)
  members, 22, 48, 59, 60, 62, 70–2, 113, 138, 141, 172, 177, 214–21
  therapy, 219
  values, 218
fidelity, 74, 241, 249
flashbacks, 33
formulation
  5 Ps, 100, 146
  CBT, 98, 99, 256, 260
  hot cross bun, 99
  psychological, 21, 217
  team-based, 233
Functional Communication Training, 3

G

gender-specific, 171
Glasgow Anxiety Scale, 70, 77
Glasgow Depression Scale, 70, 77, 95
graded exposure, 23, 104, 112, 113, 128–30
grounding techniques, 187, 203
group(s)
  cohesion, 158
  disempowered, 214
  dynamics, vii, 159, 168, 170, 173, 225
  therapists, 159, 162, 165, 171, 173, 174, 176
  therapy, 42, 157–62, 167, 177, 225
guided
  discovery, 241, 244
  self-help, 12

H

Hassle Logs, 172
health
  inequalities, 32, 62, 239, 247
  promotion, 168, 238
homework, 39, 60, 93, 111, 113, 114, 119, 130, 138, 203, 213, 217, 222, 241, 242
humour, 35, 47

I

Increasing Access for Psychological Therapies (IAPT), 32, 246, 247
inequalities, 181
inferences, 17, 86, 91, 93, 119
inferential beliefs, 45
information processing, 11, 15, 22
informed consent, 169
inquiry process, 187, 193
interactional analysis, 39
interpersonal, 18, 21, 24, 25, 62, 68, 99, 121, 140, 141, 144, 158, 160, 161, 176, 193, 257
interventions
  behavioural, 35
  ethical and psychological principles, 173, 225
  group, 158, 159, 163, 166, 168, 172, 173, 176, 223, 225
  individual, 159
  low intensity, 223
  manualised, 132, 249, 250
  pharmacological, 35
  psychosocial, 35
  psychotherapeutic, 158
Inventory of Interpersonal Problems, 71

IPA, 161
IQ, 14, 34

J
job
  description, 222
  satisfaction, 227

K
Key-worker, 159
kindness, 186, 188, 193, 204, 205

L
language
  comprehension, 38, 39
  expression, 38, 39
  simple, 43, 141, 155
lay therapist, 159, 223, 227, 248, 249
learned helplessness, 40, 41, 49
learning history, 40, 41
literacy, 17, 41, 65, 72–4, 76, 80, 81, 104, 118, 130, 168, 173, 246
loss, 19, 103, 168, 221, 230, 232

M
mainstreaming agenda, 35
manual, 55, 134, 159, 195, 199, 246–9
Manualised Group Intervention Checklist, 249
measures
  follow-up, 169
  post-, 169
  pre-, 169

memory, 5, 13, 16, 41, 65, 66, 71, 72, 87, 137–9, 154, 155, 170, 174, 183, 195, 202, 243, 256
metacognitive shift, 38
metacompetent adherence, 25, 31, 47, 219
mindful movement, 186, 200, 201
mindfulness, vi, vii, 166, 181–208, 237
Mindfulness Based Cognitive Therapy (MBCT), 181, 182, 184–6, 188, 193, 202, 207
Mindfulness Based Stress Reduction (MBSR), 182, 195
mindfulness of breathing, 186, 201
mindfulness of eating, 186
mindfulness storyboard, 198
modelling, 46, 160
motivation, 39–41, 45, 56, 58, 72, 79, 82, 97, 104, 113, 114, 118, 123, 128, 130, 149, 160, 164, 170, 217
multi-disciplinary teams (MDTs), 89, 233

N
narrative therapy, 219
National Institute for Health and Care Excellence (NICE) guidelines, 32, 183
negative automatic thoughts (NATs), 18, 38, 43
negative triad, 11
nightmares, 33
non verbal cues, 67, 141
non-specific factors, 24, 63, 159–61
normalisation, 158
Novaco Anger Scale, 71

O

occupational therapists, 130, 231
offending, 14, 158
outcomes
   desired, 220, 226
   health, 229
   long term, 172
   measures, 70
   positive, 176, 222, 226
outreach, 37, 60–2, 100, 113, 130

P

parent(s)
   divorce, 220
   older, 216
pathological, 256
peer(s)
   relationships, 147, 153, 175, 176
   support, 175, 176, 245
perpetuating, 100, 147
person centred approach, 46
personal construct theory, 11, 78
phenomenology, 242
physical needs, 205–206
planning, 16, 41, 72, 75, 113, 169, 206, 222, 243
post-structuralism, 220
poverty, 19, 21, 34, 99, 232
power
   balance, 39
   dynamics, 220
pragmatic blending, 160
precipitating, 100, 147
predisposing, 100, 147
prerequisite skills, 44–6
present moment awareness, 187–9, 198

presenting problems, 33, 36, 81, 142, 147, 223, 256
problem solving, vi, 1, 16, 41, 112, 168, 175
process issues, 42, 161, 240, 245, 256, 258
professional(s), vi, vii, 36, 56, 58, 64, 65, 87, 95, 113, 214–16, 218, 227–31, 233, 238, 243, 245, 249, 250, 257
protective factors, 35, 65, 100, 104, 147
Provocation Index, 159
Provocation Inventory, 71
psychiatrists, 79, 231, 232
psychodynamic, 160, 176
psycho-educational, 46, 167, 182
psychological
   distress, 15, 40, 162, 213, 215, 226
   formulation, 21
   health, 221
   make up, 213
   mindedness, 35, 172
   needs, 160, 173, 177, 217, 246, 259
   therapies, 14, 32, 120, 163, 167, 238, 239, 242, 251
   understanding, 214
   well being, 5, 176, 214, 224, 229, 233
psychologists, 232
psychometric(s), 14, 161, 169
psychosis, v, 10, 14, 24, 78, 240
psychotic symptoms, 33
psychotropic medication
   contra-indicative for CBT, 231
   side effects, 230

posttraumatic disorder (PTSD), 33, 158, 163, 165
public health, 238

R

randomised controlled trial (RCT), 47, 227, 248
rating scales, 71, 73, 75–8, 249
Rational Emotive Behavioural Therapy (REBT), 13, 97
reasonable adjustments, 42, 230
reciprocity, 226, 227
recording sheets, 72, 104, 114
Reed and Clements's assessment, 66
referral, 15, 56, 59, 79, 142, 152, 170
rehearsal, 150, 152
relationships
  collaborative, 90, 241, 257
  family, 221
  intimate, 213
  reciprocal, 35, 203, 227
  sexual, 88
relaxation exercises, 164, 166, 171
remediation, 46, 49
repertory grids, 78, 79
repetition, 66, 115, 155, 195, 202
research, vi, vii, 2, 5–7, 13, 19, 43–5, 68, 78, 96, 124, 132, 134, 158, 161, 176, 183, 184, 200, 201, 206, 215, 216, 227, 228, 240, 244, 245, 248, 251, 258, 259
  qualitative, 161, 176
  quantitative, 161
residential
  services, 37
  settings, 229

responsibility, 63, 155, 160, 220, 226
rigid thinking, 5, 137, 142, 146, 147, 149, 152, 154
role-play, 13, 38, 70, 76, 94, 95, 118, 119, 123, 129, 130, 145, 149, 150, 152, 154, 166, 175, 184, 198, 202, 205, 258
Rosenberg Self-Esteem Scale, 71

S

scaffolding, 24, 25, 73, 115, 118, 258
schema
  confidence, 101, 104, 114
  core, 11
  self, 11, 101
schizophrenia, 33, 230
Scottish Intercollegiate Guidelines Network (SIGN) guidelines, 183
self
  care, 220
  efficacy, 45, 88, 125, 138
  esteem, 32, 71, 101, 104, 127, 160, 169, 194
  perception, 34, 78–82, 93, 101, 146, 147
  regulation, 16, 40, 41, 87, 183, 201
  talk, 16
self compassion, 184, 193, 194, 199
self monitoring, 67, 71, 72, 75, 117, 138, 143
self regulation, 16, 40, 41, 87, 183, 201
sensory focused exercises, 199
sensory integration, 231

service(s)
　deficiencies, 231
　delivery model, 37
　development, 227
　health, 2, 35–7, 132, 182, 217, 223, 228, 245, 246
　managers, 172
　principles, 218
　provision, 167
　social, 152, 167, 169, 214, 229–31
　statutory, 221
sessions
　follow-up, 59, 176, 184
　group, 164, 170, 171, 173, 175, 176, 186, 222
　one to one, vii, 5, 61
　training, 173, 225
sexual
　abuse, 218
　activity, 218
　education, 218
　freedom, 218
　offending, 14, 33, 158, 162
sexuality, 95, 218, 220, 255
siblings, 215, 217
situational competence, 48
social
　anxiety, 10, 13, 17, 122, 192
　change, 214
　constructionist, 161
　deprivation, 39
　exclusion, 21, 34
　isolation, 99
　role valorisation, 218
　services, 152, 167, 169, 214, 229, 231
　settings, 23, 192, 214
　workers, 153, 220, 231
social care, 37, 58, 65, 88, 89, 101, 127, 128, 202, 229, 249

social cognitive, 66, 68, 78, 144
social information processing, 68
social model of disability, 238
Socratic questioning, 12, 25, 117
soles of the feet meditation, 189, 195, 207
Special Needs Schools, 167
speech and language therapists (SALTs), 231
staff-training, 173
standardised assessment, 70, 71, 89
stepped care model, 250
stigma, 34, 101, 102, 124–7, 243
storyboard, 68–70, 144, 149, 150, 198, 199
strategies
　constructive, 220
　coping, 33, 43, 123, 152, 162, 167, 176
　effective, 43, 149, 175, 214, 220
　preventative, 168, 213
stress, vi, 34, 42, 92, 154, 164, 183, 197, 216, 227
supervision, 37, 159, 223, 227, 228, 239, 244, 245, 247, 248, 250, 259
support
　networks, 65, 143, 153, 213
　workers, 23, 37, 48, 62, 72, 89, 95, 97, 99, 113, 117, 164, 165, 171–3, 221–6, 228, 230
symbolic interactionist theory, 22, 23, 127
symbols, 73, 75, 141

T

Thematic Analysis, 161
theory of mind, 94, 120

therapeutic
 alliance, 42
 change, 42, 109–34, 166
 competencies, 47, 109
 dialogue, 62, 115–18, 258
 distain, 3
 goals, 78, 102, 146, 218, 220
 process, 5, 23, 24, 39, 56, 59, 62, 213, 217, 222, 224, 226, 227, 249, 258
 relationship, 23, 24, 42, 45, 63, 116, 127, 139, 154, 158, 166, 217, 227, 256
third wave therapies, 5, 181, 195, 207
thought diaries, 38
three systems model, 193
tick box, 77, 114
training
 communication, 3, 62, 228, 242, 243
 lack of, 227
 as an ongoing process, 228
 opportunities, 228
 poor, 229
 in the workplace, 228
transdiagnostic, 133
trauma, 14, 19, 33, 158, 162–5, 167, 193, 194, 232
trauma-focused cognitive behavioural therapy (TF-CBT), 163–5, 169, 224

turn taking, 38, 88, 141
 difficulties, 140, 141

U
unconscious, 109
underlying assumptions, 218

V
values, 10, 17, 18, 25, 61, 86–8, 100, 109, 118, 127, 128, 162, 163, 170, 188, 218, 226, 251, 256, 260
verbal communication, 3, 46
visual materials, 90, 141
visual media, 46

W
weighing scales, 119, 151
well-being, 6, 16, 25, 117, 214, 216, 224, 227, 229–31
work, 231

Z
Zippy's Friends, 167, 168
zone of proximal development, 24, 258

The manufacturer's authorised representative in the EU is Springer Nature Customer Service Centre GmbH, Europaplatz 3, 69115 Heidelberg, Germany. If you have any concerns regarding our products, please contact ProductSafety@springernature.com

Printed and bound by CPI Group (UK) Ltd, Croydon, CR0 4YY
23/03/2026
02076673-0004